PREFACE.

A FEW years since, several of my personal friends, having expressed a wish to have some instructions concerning the diseases of females, and the conduct to be observed during pregnancy, labour, and confinement; and also directions for the management of new-born infants, in accordance with the principles of our school; I was induced to prepare for the press, a short treatise on the Homœopathic treatment of the diseases of females and children. Several subjects and diseases were introduced which were not contained in works published before that time.

The first edition is now exhausted, and the call for a second, is accompanied with a request to include the general diseases incident to childhood and youth.

Those additions have been made in the present edition, and the dose, repetition, and mode of administration, affixed to the indications for each remedy.

The book is not written for criticism, but in the hope that it may be useful in the treatment of the various diseases mentioned, it is offered to the public.

AUTHOR.

Philadelphia, January 2d, 1854.

DISEASES

OF

FEMALES AND CHILDREN:

AND THEIR

HOMŒOPATHIC TREATMENT.

CONTAINING ALSO,

A FULL DESCRIPTION OF THE DOSE OF EACH MEDICINE.

BY WALTER WILLIAMSON, M. D.,

PROFESSOR OF MATERIA MEDICA AND THERAPEUTICS IN THE HOMŒOPATHIC MEDICAL COLLEGE OF PENNSYLVANIA.

2d ed.

PHILADELPHIA:

PUBLISHED BY RADEMACHER & SHEEK, 239 ARCH ST.

NEW YORK: WM. RADDE.—BOSTON: OTIS CLAPP.—ST. LOUIS: J. G. WESSELHŒFT.—PITTSBURGH: J. G. BACKOFEN.—CHICAGO: D. S. SMITH, M. D.—NEW ORLEANS: D. R. LUYTIES, M. D. MANCHESTER, ENG.: H. TURNER.

1854.

Stereotyped by G. CHARLES. Printed by KING & BAIRD.

DIET.

ALLOWED.

Pure water, toast water, gum arabic water, weak black tea, cocoa and plain chocolate.

Panada, gruel, arrow-root, tapioca, sago, and farina; fresh milk, sweet cream, good butter, and soft boiled eggs ; water crackers, light bread and plain biscuit, at least one day old; puddings made of wheat, rye, corn, rice, or stale bread.

Potatoes, tomatoes, beets, peas, beans, squashes, cauliflower and asparagus.

Beef, mutton, good ham, farm-yard fowls, small game, and oysters ; fresh perch, rock fish, and small creek fish ; salted shad and salmon.

Soup of beef, mutton, and farm-yard fowls ; thickened with rice, barley, or wheat flour ; and seasoned with a little salt.

Sugar, salt, and molasses in small quantities ; ripe fruit, possessing little or no acidity, in its season, and plain preserves made of the same.

If any of the above articles should disagree, on account of constitutional peculiarity or the nature of the disease, they ought to be avoided.

FORBIDDEN.

Coffee, green tea, spiced chocolate, vinegar, lemonade, all vinous, fermented and distilled liquors, mineral waters, acids, spices, aromatics, perfumery, tobacco, snuff and segars.

All kinds of pastry, cheese, buckwheat cakes, short cakes, doughnuts, egg plant, cabbage, turnips, parsnips, carrots, onions, radishes, horse-radish, salads, celery, parsley, greens, cucumbers, pickles, highly-seasoned sauces, soups, and broths, all kinds of nuts, acid and unripe fruits.

Fresh pork, scrapple, sausages, mince pies, fried oysters, smoked meat and fish, salt mackerel, veal, turkeys, geese, ducks, lobsters, crabs, catfish, eels, &c.

All domestic medicines, herb teas, &c.; as well as the external use of camphor, hartshorn, cologne water, bay rum, vinegar, turpentine, &c.

Hot bread and warm cakes, as well as bread and cakes raised with soda, salæratus, pearl-ash, fermenting powders, &c.

Fruit, boiled vegetables, fresh fish, oysters, eggs and chicken soup, should not be eaten in cases of colic, cholera morbus, diarrhœa or dysentery.

CONTENTS.

PART I.

DISEASES OF FEMALES.

PART II.

TREATMENT OF CHILDREN.

PART III.

GENERAL DISEASES.

PART I.

DISEASES OF FEMALES.

DISEASES OF FEMALES.

THE female constitution, especially after puberty, possesses distinctive peculiarities, independent of the influence of habits and of education. And these peculiarities extend to the moral as well as the physical being. The particular organization of the female subjects her to many diseases, as well as physiological changes not of a morbid character, from which the male is exempt. The object of the present chapter is to treat of some of the most common of those diseases, derangements, and changes.

MENSTRUATION.

When this function is performed in a healthy manner, no change of consequence is perceptible in the general feelings; although increased susceptibility of the nervous system sometimes attends it. The first approach of this change is generally marked by a reserve in the manners; a more erect carriage; a change in the voice; expansion of the chest; enlargement of the breasts, &c.

The quantity differs very much in different individuals—the average quantity is perhaps from four to six ounces. When perfectly healthy it does not coagulate, and the stain is very difficult to wash out. In quite young females, or those who menstruate too soon, the quantity is generally smaller and more mixed with mucus; sometimes nearly white, and merely streaked with red. The duration of a menstrual period varies in different persons from two to seven days; the average is about five days. It usually returns with great regularity in a state of health every twenty-eight days, except in girls who menstruate precociously; and again when approaching the period of its final cessation, or the change of life, as this stage is called.

The above account may be considered a brief outline of healthy menstruation, and any considerable deviation therefrom, especially if it affect the general health, should be corrected by appropriate medical treatment. Derangements of menstruation are generally referable to insufficient clothing, fault in regimen, or improper action of the mind.

TOO TARDY APPEARANCE OF THE MENSES.

The absence of this discharge alone, so long as the general health does not suffer, is not sufficient reason for the administration of medicine. It is sometimes delayed in our latitude until the eighteenth year, without any evil consequences resulting. It generally, however, occurs at the age of fourteen or fifteen years. Carefully avoid taking all nostrums, herb teas, essential oils, or other forcing medicines, for the purpose of bringing it on. But when all the visible signs of womanhood have appeared, with the mental and moral changes that usually take place at the period of puberty, and the menses do not yet show themselves, especially if periodical pains in the hips, loins and back occur, attended with a sensation of weight and fulness in the lower part of the abdomen, with bearing down, the aid of medicine may with propriety be called in to relieve the sufferer. A long catalogue of additional symptoms occasionally occurring at this period might be enumerated as calling for treatment: such as fulness about the head, giddiness, flushed face or sallowness, bleeding at the nose, buzzing in the ears, palpitation of the heart, constriction of the chest, shortness of breath on going up stairs, hardness and soreness in the breasts drawing and numbness in the lower limbs, lassitude, feeble pulse, fainting fits, hysterical symptoms, coldness of the limbs, swelling of the ankles, swelling of the abdomen, nausea, colic, constipation, leucorrhœa, &c.

The causes which impede menstruation may be very remote and obscure, or they may be immediate and apparent. As the notices of disease in the present treatise are necessarily short and confined to the most prominent points, the cases treated of under this head will be selected from those of the most frequent occurrence, and of the simpler forms. Recommending those arising from occult causes, or depending on some organic derangement, to the management of a judicious homœopathic physician.

When the general health is but slightly affected by the apparent delay of this important function, a well ordered regimen is frequently all that is necessary to bring about the "change." Let the diet be simple but nutritious; consisting of easily digestible articles in due proportion from the animal and vegetable kingdoms; avoiding compounded cookeries, high seasoning and spices, as well as the use of tea and coffee, and all stimulating drinks, such as cider, porter, beer, wine, spirits, &c. Let her pursue a regular course of exercise: such as walking in the open air in suitable weather, riding on horseback or in an open carriage; taking a share in the duties of housekeeping, &c.; being careful to avoid fatigue or excessive exercise, and exposure to a draft of air when in a state of perspiration. Sedentary habits and too close application to study are very injurious. Cultivate cheerfulness of disposition, and endeavor to promote it by choosing such pastimes as will at once amuse and divert the mind. Pay proper attention to dress—let the clothing be seasonable and changed to suit the variations of the weather; protect the feet and lower limbs against cold, and carefully avoid exposure to wet and dampness.

The medicines chiefly employed in the cases alluded to above, are—*Arsenicum*, *Belladonna*, *Bryonia*, *Cocculus*, *Cuprum*, *Lachesis*, *Lycopodium*, *Phosphorus*, *Pulsatilla*, *Sepia*, *Sulphur* and *Veratrum.*

Arsenicum, if the face is pale and swelled in the morning on rising, with swelling of the feet in the evening, and a sensation of heat in the circulation with prostration of strength.

Dose.—Three globules night and morning for a week, or until improvement takes place.

Belladonna, if bleeding of the nose, redness of the face, injected eyes with dread of light attend, or if there be a full pulse, dark redness of the face, and giddiness after stooping. Aconite may be given alternately with Belladonna.

Dose.—Four globules three times a day until relief is afforded, or the two remedies may be given in alternation.

Bryonia, if, in place of menstruation, bleeding of the nose occurs. Lachesis and Lycopodium may also be given in similar cases.

Dose.—Six globules every morning, for several mornings in succession.

Cocculus, if there should be a complication of nervous affections, contracting pinching pains in the lower part of the abdomen, with oppressed respiration and groaning.

Dose.—Six globules every night until better.

Cuprum, is indicated when the patient is threatened with spasms, or has cramps in the lower limbs, with screaming, nausea, and vomiting.

Dose.—Four globules three times a day until relief is afforded.

Lachesis, is applicable when symptoms of suffocation attend, and all the sufferings are aggravated after sleep; also, if there be fainting fits and convulsions.

Dose.—Three globules night and morning.

Phosphorus, in females of a delicate form, with light complexion and lively disposition, weak chest and a predisposition to disease of the lungs, expectoration of blood in small quantities, or dyspeptic symptoms alternating with rheumatic pains.

Dose.—Six globules every other night.

Pulsatilla, if there be pain in the abdomen and across the back, giddiness, fulness about the head and eyes, paleness of the face, with occasional flashes of heat; roaring in the ears, or partial deafness; coldness of the hands and feet, with predisposition to general coldness; hysterical symptoms, alternate laughing and crying; nausea and vomiting; sour taste in the mouth after eating; discouragement and sadness; palpitation of the heart; soreness of the breast; loss of appetite, with desire for acids, and aversion to exercise. The unpleasant sensations frequently change from one place to another, or are felt on but one side of the body at a time. She feels better during exercise, and in the open air; generally worse in the evening and before midnight, and is fatigued in the morning.

Dose.—Six globules every afternoon until improvement is evident, or until the menses make their appearance.

Sepia, if, in addition to many of the above symptoms, there should be a yellow streak across the nose and on the cheeks in the form of a saddle. It should be given at night: twice in succession.

Dose.—Four globules at night for several nights in succession.

Sulphur, if neither of the above remedies should answer the purpose, and there be a sensation of heat in the interior of the brain; great religious depression; emaciation; want of appetite, with sickness after eating; vertigo; palpitation of the heart, and shortness of breath on going up stairs, worse when standing; to be given at night, as above directed for the other remedies.

Dose.—Four globules at night as directed for Sepia.

Veratrum, if there be cold hands and feet, with a tendency to diarrhœa.

Dose.—Six globules night and morning until relieved.

CHLOROSIS, OR GREEN SICKNESS.

On account of the very common occurrence of this disease about the period of puberty in females, and the uniform attendance of suppressed or vitiated menstruation *consequent* upon it, the affection itself is frequently looked upon as the *result* of such derangement. This state of the system, however, has been witnessed in females of mature age, and even sometimes in males, having a lymphatic temperament and delicate constitution.

Any of the causes which so frequently produce derangement of the female economy may give rise to this disease. The most common exciting causes are cold and exposure to dampness; sedentary habits, want of exercise and fresh air; powerful emotions of the mind, disappointment and chagrin; errors in diet, food not sufficiently nourishing, and the too free use of acids and stimulating drinks.

As the disease under consideration is a complicated one, and one of very serious import, involving the all of health, none but a qualified physician should attempt its treatment, if the services of one can be obtained.

The medicines that are generally sufficient in this affection, are: *Bryonia*, *China*, *Conium*, *Ferrum*, *Kali carb.*, *Lycopodium*, *Natrum mur.*, *Pulsatilla*, *Sepia*, and *Sulphur*.

Bryonia, if there is congestion to the head, bleeding of the nose or oppression of the chest, chilliness in alternation with dry burning heat, tongue coated, with pressure and fullness in the region of the stomach.

Dose.—Three globules, dissolved in a teaspoonful of water, every six hours until better, and then not so often.

China, where there is much debility, with feeling of soreness and hard swelling of the thighs with pressure toward the genital organs, congestion to the head, and bloated face with protrusion of the eyes, heartburn, or vomiting of sour mucus.

Dose.—Six globules in a spoonful of water night and morning.

Conium. Abdominal spasms, with discharge of a white acrid mucus from the vagina, causing a burning sensation; nausea and vomiting, with coldness of the feet, and pain as if from soreness in the lower part of the back.

Dose.—Six globules three times a day until relief is afforded.

Ferrum metallicum. Giddiness during motion, aching pain in the stomach, countenance pale, lips pale and bluish, menses scanty and flesh colored, emaciation and debility, swelling of the hands and feet, urine clear, with much chilliness.

Dose.—Three globules night and morning for a week, or until a favorable change takes place.

Kali Carbonicum, if the menses have been suppressed, and there is pain in the abdomen with soreness of the pudendum, or the menstrual discharge has an acrid pungent smell, pale greenish urine, aching in the head, with ill humor, face pale, with faint, lifeless eyes.

Dose.—Three globules twice a day for several days, and if improvement takes place, then discontinue it for a few days, and resume again if necessary.

Lycopodium, bloatedness of the abdomen; coldness of the feet, with heaviness of the limbs; urine dark and burning, with sandy sediment; sleep restless and full of fancies; heaviness in the head;

face pale, with blueness around the eyes; and swelling of the limbs.

Dose.—Six globules every morning for a week, dissolved in a tablespoonful of water, and if no change takes place, another remedy must be selected according to the symptoms.

Natrum Muriaticum, in obstinate cases, when there is retention of the menstrual discharges, or profuse leucorrhœa, with discharge of a transparent white, thick mucus, or greenish leucorrhœa, with yellowness of the face, headache, and congestion of blood to the head.

Dose.—Six globules night and morning; in other respects the same as Lycopodium.

Pulsatilla is one of our most prominent remedies in this disease, especially if it is attended with derangement of the digestive organs; often shifting from one place to another; complexion sallow; difficult breathing; coldness of the hands and feet; nausea, with inclination to vomit; acrid leucorrhœa, with discharge of thick, white mucus; cough, with expectoration of thick mucus; periodical expectoration of dark clotted blood; hunger, with aversion to food. It is best adapted to females of a mild disposition.

Dose.—Four globules in a dessertspoonful of water night and morning for a week, then pause eight days, after which the course may, if necessary, be repeated as before.

Sepia, discharge of yellowish leucorrhœa with itching in the vagina; soreness and redness of the labia; oppression of breathing, with rush of blood to the head; violent headache, as if the head would burst; urine turbid, with brick-dust sediment; pain in the small of the back, with pain in the thighs as if bruised.

Dose.—The same as directed for Pulsatilla.

Sulphur is one of the most valuable remedial agents that can be employed in this disease, especially if the patient is afflicted with any constitutional taint; it is especially indicated if there should be pressive pain in the back of the head, extending to the nape of the neck, with determination of blood and humming in the head; distension of the stomach and abdomen; irregular bowels; breathing difficult; great fatigue, especially of the limbs; great tendency to take cold; sadness and melancholy, with frequent weeping.

Dose.—Six globules night and morning, until amelioration or change takes place.

SUPPRESSION OF THE MENSES.

By suppression of the menses, is understood the suspension or temporary cessation of this discharge, after it has been well established, by some incidental cause. Cold is the most common cause of this obstruction, as it is the one to which females are the most liable, on account of the little care they take of themselves at the menstrual period. Sudden and powerful emotions of the mind, particularly grief and despondency, may also produce it, but next after the first mentioned cause is the malicious practice of eating pickles, drinking vinegar, and putting the feet in cold water during the flow, for the purpose of aresting it. Disease of the chest and of the liver, rheumatism, and inflammation of the organs concerned, may also give rise to suppression. Any of these causes may act so as to produce the result during the flow, when the menses are about to appear, or during the interval. If the menses are suddenly suppressed during the flow or just as they are about to appear, especially if cold be the cause, the symptoms are apt to be much more violent than as if the obstructing cause were applied in the interval. In the worst cases are seen frightful attacks of spasmodic pains in the stomach and bowels, often attended with retching to vomit, headache, flushed face, wild delirium, convulsions, hysteria, palpitation of the heart, difficulty of breathing, &c. This state of things is sometimes followed by fever and local inflammations. When suppression of the menses is the effect of causes operating in the interval, the evil consequences do not arise so suddenly, nor are they so alarming; yet, after the lapse of two or three months, the enfeebled state of health evinces the no less certain result. The subject becomes pale, languid, and debilitated; loses her appetite and ambition; looks sickly and dejected; is affected with swelling of the feet and ankles; nervous symptoms set in; palpitation of the heart, shortness of breath, flatulency, &c., and leucorrhœa winds up the unhappy train. In persons predisposed to consumption and some other serious diseases, suppression is particularly prejudicial and demands the earliest attention.

The medicines generally required in the treatment of this affection are *Aconite*, *Bryonia*, *Pulsatilla*, *Sepia* and *Sulphur*. But *Belladonna*, *Chamomilla*, *Graphites*, *Kali carb.*, *Lycopodium*, *Platina* and *Veratum* are sometimes necessary.

Aconite, if the suppression be the result of the direct application of cold, and be attended by congestion to the head or chest; redness of the cheeks; sickness, faintness or giddiness on rising from a recumbent position; shooting and beating pains in the head, with delirium or stupefaction; fulness of the pulse; impatience—worse from motion; cold gives relief, but heat aggravates the sufferings.

Dose.—Six globules every six hours in a tablespoonful of water until relieved.

Bryonia, if there be swimming in the head, with heaviness and pressure towards the forehead, worse after stooping, and aggravated by motion; bleeding of the nose; dry cough; shivering during the pains; heat on the head; pain in the pit of the stomach after eating; bitter and sour eructations; regurgitation of food after eating with a good appetite; constipation; drawing pains in the lower part of the abdomen; pain in the back; the sufferings are increased by motion and by touching; this remedy is particularly adapted to unmarried females.

Dose.—Three globules in a spoonful of water at intervals of twelve hours, until decided amelioration or change for the better.

Pulsatilla is the principal remedy in this disease, especially when it has been caused by exposure to dampness or cold air, and the subject have an amiable disposition with a tendency to sadness and tears; the headache is generally on one side only, with shooting pains extending to the face, ears, and teeth; palpitation of the heart; suffocation; coldness of the hands and feet; flashes of heat; nausea and vomiting; tendency to diarrhœa; pressure in the lower part of the abdomen; frequent urination, and leucorrhœa.

Dose.—Three globules in a spoonful of water night and morning for a week, (unless change should sooner occur,) then wait eight days, after which it may, if necessary, be repeated as before, until relief is obtained.

Sepia, is also a very important remedy, especially in females of a delicate constitution and sallow complexion; the symptoms are often relieved by exercise, and aggravated by rest; great liability to take cold; disposed to melancholy; morning headache; throbbing in the head; vertigo; bearing down in the lower part of the abdomen, with heat and sensitiveness; leucorrhœa; colic; pains in the limbs, as if they had been beaten; pain in the loins.

Dose.—Six globules in a tablespoonful of water every other day, continuing the same for some time, until amelioration takes place.

Sulphur, if the person has been subject to eruptions; disposition to stiffness in all parts of the body; want of strength; faintness; exhaustion from conversation; sensitiveness to the open air; disposition to sleep; the heat of the bed aggravates the pains at night; confusion of the head; vertigo on rising up; headache on one side or over the eyes, or in the back part of the head, extending to the back of the neck; heat in the head; heaviness of the head; dimness of sight; sourness of the stomach; waterbrash; pressure in the stomach; voracious appetite; constipation, with ineffectual efforts at stool; abdominal pains; leucorrhœa, with itching; pain in the loins; weariness and fatigue in the limbs.

Dose.—The same as directed for Sepia.

BELLADONNA, if it should occur without any particular exciting cause, and be attended with fulness of blood, and violent throbbing of the arteries of the head and neck.

Dose.—Three globules every twelve hours, until amelioration or change takes place.

Chamomilla, great sensitiveness of the abdomen, pain in the small of the back, extending down the thigh, diarrhœa, with greenish or white stool, desire to vomit, yellow coated tongue, and bitter taste in the mouth.

Dose.—Six globules night and morning.

Graphites, in cases where there is either total suppression, or where the discharge is very scanty, the blood black, or watery and pale, headache, nausea, pain in the chest, swelling of the feet and legs.

Dose.—Six globules night and morning.

Kali Carbonicum, when the oppression has occurred in an apparently healthy female, and the arrest of discharge can be traced to no special cause.

Dose.—The same as of Graphites.

Lycopodium, where suppression is caused by fright, attended with dryness of the vagina, bloatedness of the abdomen, heaviness of the limbs, chilliness, nausea and swelling of the feet.

Dose.—Six globules night and morning.

Platina, painful pressure towards the genitals with drawing headache, drawing in the abdomen before the menses make their appearance, with cutting pain and cramps, great sensitiveness of the parts.

Dose.—Six globules dissolved in a tumbler half full of water, and take a teaspoonful of the solution every four or six hours, according to circumstances.

Veratrum, if menstruation is preceded by vertigo; bleeding at the nose; great thirst; buzzing in the ears; pain in all the limbs; colic affecting the whole abdomen; redness and heat of the face; palpitation of the heart; pain in the small of the back; heaviness of the limbs.

Dose.—Four globules three times a day until relief is obtained, or the symptoms require another remedy.

If menstruation has been checked by fright, vexation, or other emotions of the mind, give *Aconite*, *Coffea*, or *Lycopodium*.

If the suppression have connection with rheumatic pains about the shoulders and chest, and the subject be predisposed to consumption, send for a physician without delay.

PAINFUL MENSTRUATION.

Women are liable to this disease during every part of their life, between the commencement and the cessation of menstruation. Cold, and the improper treatment of other diseases, are the most prolific sources of this derangement. The pain sometimes begins several hours or even days before the flow commences, at other times the evacuation comes on regularly and continues for a few hours, then diminishes, or ceases entirely, with a great deal of suffering. The pains may continne for a longer or shorter period; frequently under appropriate treatment the flow returns, and continues to the end of the period without interruption; sometimes the pains continue to the end of the period without shortening the time or lessening the quantity. At other times the pains continue until a membranous substance is expelled, and a healthy discharge continues, or the evacuation ceases with the expulsion of the membranous body. In some cases through sympathy, the breasts become sensitive, tumid, and occasionally extremely painful. The pains of difficult menstruation are of two kinds, viz.: the intermitting expulsive pains resembling those of labor, and the constant aching pains in the loins, hips and limbs, like those which often precede regular menstruation.

The remedies are: *Aconite*, *Belladonna*, *Calcarea*, *Chamomilla*, *Cocculus*, *Coffea*, *Nux vomica*, *Pulsatilla*, and *Veratrum*.

Aconite, if febrile symptoms are present, such as accelerated pulse; thirst; quick, hurried breathing; headache; restlessness; congestion to the head or chest; faintness and giddiness—worse on motion.

Dose.—Dissolve twelve pellets in six teaspoonsful of water, and take a teaspoonful every hour until the sufferings are relieved.

Belladonna, if the pains precede the flow, with violent congestion to the head, and confusion of sight; frightful visions; screaming; disposition to bite and tear everything; redness and bloatedness of the face; pain in the back; strong bearing down in the lower part of the abdomen, as if the parts would fall out.

Dose.—Six globules dissolved in a teaspoonful of water, and repeated every four or six hours until better.

Calcarea carb., if there be boring headache, which is aggravated by every moral emotion; coldness on the head; toothache; breasts swollen and painful; colic, with shiverings; cuttings in the abdomen; leucorrhœa; spasmodic pains in the loins. After the period is past, if the membranous substance spoken of above should have been discharged, give a dose of Calc. on two successive evenings, and again, four or five days before the return of the next menstrual period, give two doses more in the same way.

Chamomilla may be given, if the pains resemble labor pains, with pressure from the small of the back towards the front of the abdomen and downwards; colic, with tenderness of the abdomen when touched; discharge of a dark color and coagulated.

Dose.—Four globules every two hours, until the pain is relieved.

Cocculus, if there be abdominal spasms; flatulency; nausea and faintness; pressive colic, and cramps in the chest.

Dose.—Six globules every four hours, until the pains are alleviated or the symptoms require another remedy.

Coffea, if there be great nervous excitement, and anguish with the sufferings; exceedingly painful colic, with fullness and pressure in the bowels, with spasms which extend to the chest; delirium; wringing of the hands; grinding of the teeth; screaming; coldness over the whole body; numbness and stiffness; groaning and difficulty of breathing.

Dose.—Put twenty globules in six teaspoonsful of water, and take a teaspoonful every four hours.

Nux vomica relieves the writhing pains in the abdomen, when accompanied with nausea; pain as if bruised in the bones in front; spasms in the womb with pressure downwards, and heat; nausea and fainting; restlessness; stitches in the right side; frequent desire to urinate. Nux vom. is indicated when the menses are preceded by drawing pains in the muscles of the back of the neck, and in excitable or passionate persons.

Dose.—Six globules three times a day, until improvement takes place.

Pulsatilla will remove a heaviness resembling a stone in the abdomen, with violent pressure in the lower part, and in the small of the back, attended with drawing and numbness down the thighs; vomiting of sour mucus; shiverings, with paleness of the face; pressure to stool, with ineffectual efforts; frequent desire to pass water, and leucorrhœa.

Dose.—Four globules dissolved in a tablespoonful of water every six hours during the discharge, until improvement takes place.

Veratrum, when the menses are preceded by headache and attended with diarrhœa; excessive weakness; humming in the ears; constrictive sensation in the throat; icy coldness of the nose, hands, and feet.

Dose.—Six globules every four or six hours, until decided improvement or another remedy is required.

MENSTRUATION TOO SOON.

Belladonna, when the evacuation comes on before the time, is too copious, and is of a bright red color; discharge of fetid coagulæ; nocturnal sweat on the chest; thirst; confusion of the sight; beating headache; puffiness of the face; colic, and violent bearing down pains.

Dose.—Six globules two or three times a day, according to circumstances.

Calcarea carb. is appropriate, when the evacuation is preceded by swelling and sensitiveness of the breasts, headache, colic, shiverings and leucorrhœa; during the flow there are cuttings in the abdomen, toothache, bearing down, leucorrhœa, and enlargement of the veins.

Dose.—Four globules night and morning.

Ignatia, is very effectual where the menses return every two weeks, and are attended with hysterical symptoms; nausea and fainting; general chilliness; paleness of the face; failing of the sight; the patient cannot bear the light or noise; the abdomen is distended and hard; the pains are of the cramp-like compressing kind.

Dose.—Six globules twice a day.

Ipecacuanha is suitable, where the patient is excessively weak, uneasy, and has a dislike to all food; the discharge copious, bright red, and coagulated.

Dose.—Four globules three times a day, dissolved in a teaspoonful of water.

Natrum mur. should be given, when the monthly period is preceded by moroseness and irritability; the evacuation is too profuse, and continues too long; is attended with sadness, headache, and an inclination to lie down.

Dose.—Dissolve about twenty globules in a tumbler half full of water, and take a teaspoonful every four hours.

MENSTRUATION TOO LATE.

Kali carb. may be given, when there is constant bearing down, and still the menses do not appear, in young girls.

Dose.—Four globules three times a day until relief is obtained.

Lachesis, when the commencement of the flow is attended with violent pains in the small of the back, and subsequent spasms in the abdomen, and beatings in the head.

Dose.—Three globules, repeated at intervals of from four to six hours.

Phosphorus, if the patient has a delicate form; is predisposed to disease of the chest, and is troubled with dyspeptic symptoms; during menstruation, lancinating headache, spitting of small portions of blood, shiverings, lassitude and fever.

Dose.—Four globules night and morning.

Pulsatilla, where the menses are very irregular, sometimes coming too soon, at other times too late, and frequently too feebly; sometimes the discharge is too dark or mixed with mucus, again it is pale and watery; the sufferings also are various: nausea and vomitings, shiverings and paleness of the face, shooting pains, bearing down, constipation, &c., are frequently met with before, during, and after the period.

Dose.—Six globules twice a day, commencing several days before the expected arrival of the monthly period, and continuing it until the discharge has been fully established.

Sulphur is frequently necessary when other remedies fail, and where sick-headache precedes, attends, or follows menstruation. The reader is referred to the preceding sections on "tardy appearance" and "suppression" for many of the symptoms of this important medicine.

Dose.—Dissolve twelve globules in six teaspoonsful of water, and take a teaspoonful every three hours until relief is obtained.

MENSTRUATION TOO SCANT.

The remedies recommended for this particular irregularity, are: *Kali carbonicum*, *Lachesis*, *Nux vomica*, *Pulsatilla*, and *Sulphur*.

Inasmuch as the characteristic symptoms of these remedies are to be found in the preceding sections of this chapter, it is not necessary to repeat them here. The reader is respectfully referred to them there. The remedy which corresponds most acurately with the whole group of symptoms, is always the most appropriate one.

Administration, the same as in the preceding article.

MENSTRUATION TOO COPIOUS.

Belladonna, when the catamenia are too copious, and return too soon, with violent pressure downwards, as if something would escape, accompanied with pain in the small of the back; where the immoderate flow has been caused by exertion, or lifting something during the period. Arn., also, may be given when that is the cause. For other symptoms of Bell., see what is said under it when the menses return too soon.

Dose.—Six globules two or three times a day, according to circumstances.

Calcarea carb., after other remedies apparently well adapted to the case have been given without effect, give Calc. carb. for two mornings in succession at the next period. See some of the symptoms of this remedy under "Menstruation too soon."

Dose.—Twelve globules dissolved in half a tumbler of water, and a teaspoonful given every two or three hours, as the circumstances require.

Chamomilla will prove beneficial if the discharge is dark and clotted; flowing at intervals, accompanied by pain and dull griping, which passes from the small of the back towards the abdomen; to which symptoms may be added, thirst, coldness of the extremities and fainting.

Dose.—Six globules three times a day until amelioration or change.

China, sallowness; general weakness, with great tendency to perspire; dulness; swelling of the lower extremities; confusion of the head, with buzzing in the ears; faintness; the discharge may be either watery, or coagulated, gushing out at intervals, accompanied with cramplike pains in the lower part of the abdomen.

Dose.—The same as directed for Chamomilla.

Ipecacuanha, where the discharge is profuse and continued; attended with paleness, thirst, and constant desire to lie down, with great prostration.

Dose.—Three globules every four hours until improvement manifests itself.

Nux vomica, when menstruation is too copious, and returns before the twenty-eighth day; when it lasts longer than four days, stops and returns.

In such cases allow no coffee, wine, cider or brandy; no mince pies, or any thing stimulating, for several months.

Dose.—Six globules night and morning until decided amelioration.

MENSTRUATION TOO SHORT.

Most of the remedies mentioned under menstruation "too soon" and "too scant" may be given with advantage in this aberration, when the attending symptoms correspond. When the period of menstruation is rendered too short by accidental causes, look under "suppression" for the remedy.

Bryonia, *Lachesis*, *Phosphorus*, *Platina* and *Pulsatilla* are the principal remedies in this irregularity.

Bryonia, pain and uneasiness in the abdomen, as if the menses would appear; suppression of the menses, or violent pain in the back and limbs, and headache during menstruation; constipation, with hard, dry stool.

Dose.—Four globules three times a day until improvement takes place, or the symptoms require another remedy.

Lachesis, menstruation scanty and delayed; before menstruation vertigo and headache; violent pain in the abdomen during menstruation, with beating in the head; costiveness, with burning in the abdomen.

Dose.—Six globules three times a day until amelioration or change.

Phosphorus, menses too early and scanty, or too late, with pain in the back and abdomen, as if bruised; stitches from the vagina to the uterus; frequent desire to urinate previous to, and after the menses; coldness of the hands and feet.

Dose.—Six globules two or three times a day according to circumstances.

Platina, cramps upon the appearance of the menses; great sensitiveness of the parts, or the menses appear too early; anxiety in the abdomen, with pain in the small of the back, as if broken.

Dose.—Six globules night and morning, dissolved in a teaspoonful of water.

Pulsatilla, before the menses, chilliness and yawning; during the menses, pain in the stomach, chilliness and paleness of the face, with urging to stool; pain in the small of the back, extending down the thighs, with discharge of thick, dark, clotted, or else pale and watery blood, flowing by fits and starts.

Dose.—Four globules three or four times a day until relief is obtained.

MENSTRUATION TOO LONG.

Aconite, when there are congestions to different parts of tho body with shooting pains, especially about the heart and in the head; full and hard pulse; desire to be in the cool air; the patient is worse in a warm room; the discharge is bright red, and for the most part fluid, but coagulates readily.

Dose.—Six globules twice a day, for several days in succession during the period, and to be repeated several days previous to the next menstrual period.

China, paleness of the face; dark-colored under the eyes; obscuration of sight, or black spots before the eyes; roaring in the ears; pulsation in the head and neck; nocturnal headache; sleeplessness or disturbed sleep; nervous excitability; frequent desire to pass water; pains like labor; weakness and heaviness in the limbs; swelling of the feet.

Dose.—Six globules night and morning, dissolved in a tablespoonful of clear water.

Ignatia is serviceable if the dischage continues too long; and the next period is attended with hysterics, yawning, and choking.

Dose.—The medicine should be given on the fourth day of menstruation, and repeated in a day or two, and repeated again on the fourth day of the next menstrual period.

Nux vomica, when the menses return too soon, and continue too long; giddiness, constipation, nausea and faintness; the symptoms are generally worse in the morning; dragging about the loins, with bearing down in the pelvis; cramp-like pains in the abdomen, extending downwards to the thighs.

Dose.—Dissolve twelve globules in half a tumblerful of water, and take a teaspoonful every three hours until relief is obtained.

Platina, discharge thick and black, or slimy; pressure on the lower parts, with increased sensibility; menses too early, with diarrhœa, or profuse flow with drawing pains in the abdomen.

Dose.—Four globules dissolved in a teaspoonful of water, three times a day.

Sulphur will frequently change this state of the system, by giving a few doses of it after menstruation is over, and repeating it again a few days before the next period.

CESSATION OF THE MENSES.

The "change of life," or the "critical stage," as the period of the decline of the menses is called, generally occurs at or about the age of forty-five years. With ladies who have indulged themselves at the table and been fond of their ease, generally this change is apt to take place a little earlier; while with those who have led more industrious and even laborious lives, it may not come quite so soon. It sometimes occurs as early as thirty-six, and even earlier; and, on the other hand, it has been postponed in some instances until the woman has passed fifty, and even much later.

When this period of life is approaching, the menses become more or less irregular, both as to the time of their recurrence and the quantity discharged—they may either return too soon, or the interval be more protracted than usual. The quantity discharged may likewise vary from the regular amount—be very small by itself, or largely mixed with mucus, or be very profuse, amounting to a true hemorrhage. The flow frequently appears suddenly, at an unexpected moment, continues for an hour or two, and then stops, without any of the ordinary symptoms of suppression following.

Sometimes the progressive course of this change in the female economy is so gradual, and free from constitutional disturbance, that the woman passes through it before she is aware of her altered condition; until she realizes that her menses have ceased, and with them many of the frailties incidental to menstruation have disappeared. Her health is confirmed, and frequently she becomes more fleshy than she ever was before.

Others, less fortunate, are afflicted with vertigo, headache, flashes of heat, nervousness, paleness and debility; frequent passage of limpid urine in large quanties, or high colored in small quantities; pain in the lower part of the abdomen, back and hips, running down the thighs with a kind of creeping sensation; heat in the lower part of the stomach and back; piles are apt to be troublesome, and sometimes take on a vicarious office; swelling of the lower limbs; tumidity of the abdomen, which subsides from time to time without the ordinary symptoms of flatulency. Pruritus (violent itching of the private parts) is not uncommon at this period.

Not every case of slight irregularity at this period of life should be interfered with by medicine, especially if the discharge be diminishing in quantity. A well ordered regimen, however, is important in every case—the diet should be simple and digestible, consisting chiefly of vegetable articles; total abstinence from everything stimulating should be strictly observed; exercise in the open air in suitable weather; bathing, and the use of the flesh brush, should be duly attended to. Sleeping in heated rooms should generally be avoided, and a matrass is better than a feather bed. In many instances it would be proper to wear flannel or silk next the skin. In all cases avoid unnecessary exposure, and guard against the injurious effects of the common vicissitudes of the weather, by suitable attention to dress.

Tonics, and the so-called strengthening medicines, are always injurious at this period, and therefore should be assiduously avoided.

REMEDIES. *Lachesis*, *Pulsatilla*, *Bryonia*, *Cocculus*, *Ignatia*, *Sepia*, and *Sulphur*.

Lachesis, scanty, delaying menses, with increased leucorrhœa, or if the menses are too profuse, attended with vertigo and headache; or lacerating pain in the abdomen, with costiveness.

Dose.—Four globules every third night, or it may be used in alternation with Pulsatilla, with much benefit.

Pulsatilla, suppression of the menses, with nausea and vomiting, chilliness, coldness of the feet, heaviness in the abdomen as if from a stone, fullness of the face, pressure in the bladder and rectum, burning pain in the abdomen.

Dose.—The same as directed for Lachesis.

Bryonia, pinching in the abdomen as if the menses would appear; suppression of the menses with bleeding at the nose, lacerating pain in the limbs and small of the back, with discharge of dark red blood.

Dose.—Six globules every night, dissolved in a teaspoonful of clear water.

Cocculus, suppression of the menses, with spasms in the abdomen, anguish, oppression of breathing, menstruation painful, with discharge of coagulated blood.

Dose.—Four globules every other night until amelioration or change.

Ignatia, menstruation scanty, with discharge of black coagulated blood, which has a putrid odor, abdominal spasms, heaviness and heat in the head, languor and faintness.

Dose.—Twelve globules dissolved in three tablespoonfuls of water, and a teaspoonful every six hours.

Sepia, before the appearance of the menses, violent colic with faintness; the discharges are scanty, shuddering over the whole body, pain in the limbs as if bruised, abdominal spasms, with pressing downwards.

Dose.—The same as directed for Ignatia.

Sulphur, burning as if in the uterus, menses too late, with pain in the abdomen and small of the back, thirst and dry tongue during the menses, discharge of bloody mucus from the vagina.

Dose.—Four globules dissolved in a teaspoonful of water twice a day, until improvement takes place.

LEUCORRHŒA.

This disease (frequently called "Whites") consists of a discharge of unhealthy mucus from the private parts, and is most liable to affect females between the age of puberty and the final cessation of the menses. Occasionally we observe it in little children, and sometimes also in women who have passed the change of life.

Women of a nervous temperament, with a relaxed habit of body, weak chest, and hereditary predisposition to it, are the most frequent subjects of this disease. The exciting causes of this complaint generally, are difficult labors; irregularity of the menses; the employment of purgative medicines; tight lacing; late hours; the immoderate use of tea, coffee, and spices; limited exercise; and sometimes the neglect of necessary ablutions. In children, the most common exciting causes are neglect of cleanliness, seat worms, and the local application of some irritating matter. Those who are subject to it at all, are liable to have the discharge most abundant before and after menstruation, and during pregnancy. The secretion may be small or very abundant, and may vary just as much in quality as it does in quantity; in the beginning, it frequently seems to be nothing more than an increase of healthy transparent mucus, but after a while it assumes a more dense consistency, and gelatinous appearance, or becomes thin, milky and acrid; after longer continuance it may become purulent, and acquire a yellow color; it is often greenish, and sometimes has a brownish hue. The discharge does not always pass away continuously, but often irregularly, by emissions.

After this discharge has continued for a longer

or shorter time, the concomitant symptoms make their appearance: such as constant pain in the back and loins; bearing down in the abdomen; aching in the hips; coldness of the extremities; paleness of the face; dejection of spirits; loss of appetite; eructations; nervous symptoms; neuralgies, &c.

Leucorrhœa is so often complicated with serious diseases of the womb and adjacent parts, that the best interests of the sufferer require the earliest attention to its treatment, and the most diligent use of the means calculated to remove it. Many now mourn with fruitless grief over their unfortunate neglect of this disease in its incipient and more manageable state. On the first intimation of the approach of the complaint, the subject of it should endeavor to correct the predisposing causes, and, as far as in her power lies, avoid all the exciting causes.

The remedies recommended in this place are: *Aconite*, *Calcarea carb.*, *Cocculus*, *Pulsatilla*, *Sepia*, and *Sulphur*.

Aconite, if the discharge be excessive, viscous, or yellowish; heat, and a sense of fullness in the parts internally: the application of anything cold gives relief, especially if the patient have been subject to acute attacks of rheumatism.

Dose.—Six globules night and morning, until improvement or change is manifested.

Calcarea carb., with itching and burning, coming on before the menses; the discharge is milky, and often passes when making water; attended with shooting through the parts, and falling of the womb; leucorrhœa after lifting; *whitish corrosive leucorrhœa of young children;* especially applicable to females of a lymphatic constitution, light complexion, and inclined to be fat, and who are subject to copious menstruation, which returns too soon.

Dose.—Four globules every morning, dissolved in a teaspoonful of water, until decided amelioration or change.

Cocculus, leucorrhœa before and after menstruation; discharge of sanguineous mucus during pregnancy; leucorrhœa like the washings of meat, with colic and flatulency.

Dose.—Three globules once a day until relief is obtained, or change should occur requiring another remedy.

Pulsatilla, when the discharge is thick, like cream; sometimes corrosive; attended with pruritus near the change of life; before, during, and after menstruation; when occasioned by fright; and, in young girls, before menstruation is well established.

Dose.—Dissolve six globules in a teaspoonful of water, night and morning, and continue it for several days, then discontinue its use for several days, after which it may be again repeated as before, if necessary.

Sepia, leucorrhœa with excoriation of the parts; bearing down; frequent urination; yellow, or greenish, fetid discharge; inflation of the abdomen; yellowness of the face—this remedy is not always admissible during pregnancy.

Dose.—Four globules every night, until improvement or change manifests itself.

Sulphur in obstinate cases of leucorrhœa, with scalding urine; whitish, or yellowish and corrosive; after repelled eruptions, or imperfectly cured rheumatism.

Dose.—Six globules two or three times a week, and continued for some length of time.

PROLAPSUS UTERI.

(Falling of the Womb.)

The chief predisposing cause of this displacement is a relaxed condition of the system, which may be natural, or induced by habits of indulgence in idleness and high living. The immediate causes of the mischief may be various; as, getting up too soon after confinement; leucorrhœa; falls; injuries from lifting heavy weights; long continued coughs; severe pukings: tight lacing, &c. An eminent physician remarked in 1831: "I will venture to say, that, of late years, since the preposterous custom of pressing the waist into as narrow a space as cords and steel springs can bring it, has been so general, there are more instances of prolapsus and leucorrhœa among *young* females than at any former period, when the abdomen was a little better accommodated with room." (Eberle.) But as fashion has changed the mode of dress considerably for the better, in this particular, since the doctor wrote the above, we may expect to see fewer cases of the diseases mentioned, arising from that cause, in the future.

The symptoms may be mild for a long time in the commencement of the disease, and be considered rather as an annoyance, than the occasion of much suffering. There is generally more or less bearing down, dragging about the groins, pain in the back and loins, pressure low down in the pelvis, a benumbing sensation shooting down the limbs, nervous feelings, with a sense of faintness, and many other exceedingly distressing symptoms. Every case does not present this long catalogue of ailments, but many cases do present them in great numbers, and in an aggravated form. In some severe cases, the woman has great difficulty in rising to her feet, and if she attempts to walk, has to lean forwards and support herself by placing her hands on her thighs. A very obscure and troublesome symptom of pain in the left side, close under the ribs, sometimes attends this disease. The sufferings are aggravated by the erect position, and nearly all of them subside after lying down.

To the above enumeration of difficulties, must be added the constant discharge of mucus, more or less unhealthy, and very generally a more abundant and frequent discharge of the menses. These two drains upon her system in conjunction with the general weakness, consequent upon uninterrupted suffering, reduces the woman's strength very much, and unless relieved, will destroy her health entirely.

For the cure of this disease, we have very frequently to employ mechanical means; namely, the "supporter," or the "pessary." But in many cases we can succeed with medicine, and a well regulated regimen. The affection itself is sometimes symptomatic of other curable diseases. Let the patient avoid the provoking causes as far as she can, adhere to the homœopathic diet, and take one of the following remedies every night for a week; namely, *Belladonna*, *Calcarea carb.*, *Nux vomica*, *Sepia*, and *Podophyllum*.

Belladonna, intense pain in the small of the back, great pressure in the lower part of the ab domem, as if its contents would issue through the genital organs, suppression of stool and urine and heaviness of the limbs.

Dose.—Six globules every night for a week, and if no improve ment, the next remedy which is most applicable to the symptoms of the case, must be used in the same manner.

Calcarea carbinica, heaviness and painful wea riness of the limbs, oppressive pains with stitches in the abdomen, contracting pain in the abdomen, drawing pain in the abdomen, extending downwards towards the genital organs.

Dose.—Four globules every night, until amelioration or change.

Nux vomica, prolapsus caused by lifting or straining, with hardness and swelling of the mouth of the womb, or burning pain, desire to urinate, constipation, with ineffectual urging to stool, attended with bearing down or forcing pains.

Dose.—Three globules in a tablespoonful of water, repeated every six hours until amelioration or change.

Sepia, painful stiffness in the region of the uterus, oppression of breathing, induration of the neck of the uterus, contractive pain in the vagina, violent pain in the abdomen, extending as far as the umbilicus.

Dose.—Four globules every night until amelioration or change.

Podophyllum pelt, pain in the region of the ovaries of a numb-aching character, fullness and soreness in the abdomen, the pain extending down the thighs.

Dose.—The same as directed for Nux vomica.

After taking one remedy and then suspending all medicine for a week or more, still adhering to the diet, if the symptoms have not abated, take one of the other remedies named in the same way, and wait as before. But if the symptoms do improve, take nothing so long as they are better, and if they return, take the last medicine once or twice more. In order to discriminate between the remedies recommended as well as you can, compare the symptoms of each remedy.

INFLAMMATION OF THE LABIA AND VAGINA.

This disease often occurs in newly-married females, and developes itself in painful, red, hard, dry, burning and sensitive swelling of the labia. Difficult and tedious labors are also frequently the cause of this inflammation; if it arises from this cause, it will readily yield to the external application of a lotion of Arnica, in the proportion of one part of Arnica tincture, to eight parts of water,—a few globules of Arnica may also be given internally. Should fever and inflammatory symptons present themselves, Aconite should be given until relief is obtained.

Dose.—Four globules every three hours.

Mercurius may be used, should the inflammation assume a lymphatic character, with much induration of the parts.

Dose.—Six globules three times a day.

Belladonna, if the disease assumes an erysipelatous appearance, with an internal feeling of fullness, tension, and burning pain.

Dose.—The same as directed for Aconite.

REGIMEN DURING PREGNANCY.

During the period of gestation a woman should consider, that her most trifling actions may exert a great influence on the future physical, and, we may add, moral and intellectual condition of a being bound to her by the most endearing ties—a being that has a right to expect from her, as its parent, so far as it lies in her power to give, a sound constitution. Therefore, to realize such an object, it becomes the duty of a mother to pay every possible attention to her diet, dress, and exercise.

DIET. With regard to diet, she should observe the greatest simplicity, and abstain from all stimulating food and drinks, as well as everything else that has a tendency to increase the irritability of the system—such as the immoderate use of coffee, tea, &c. She should also avoid taking too large an amount of nourishment of any kind; for nature seems to have instituted nausea and vomiting for the purpose, in part, of preventing excessive fullness. The occasion of pregnancy ought not to be made the apology for the free indulgence of a wayward, or a voracious appetite; as indigestion colic, and even convulsions, in some instances, have been the sad consequences of such indulgence. The unnatural use of chalk, magnesia, charcoal, roasted coffee, &c., is to be deprecated.

DRESS. The dress should be strictly suited to the season, and so arranged as not to produce unnecessary pressure on any part of the body; even the garters should be worn loosely. Tight lacing is very hurtful: it must be evident to the plainest understanding, that serious injury to the health of both mother and child must often result from a continual and forcible compression of the abdomen, while nature is at work in gradually enlarging it for the accommodation and development of the fœtus; and, no doubt, there are many who owe their deformities to the vanity or fastidiousness of their mothers.

EXERCISE. With regard to exercise, here let us say, that it is indispensibly necessary to health during the term of pregnancy. The most useful kind of exercise is *walking* in the open air; for this calls into action more of the muscles of the body than any other exercise suited to the state of pregnancy. Such exercise must not, however, interfere with the process of digestion; and, therefore, the most suitable time for it is two or three hours after a moderate dinner, or, during warm weather, towards evening—care being taken to avoid the dampness of the night air by returning home early. The passive exercise of riding in a carriage falls short of the object in view, and the violent exercise of riding on horse-back exceeds it, besides the liability to fright and accident which besets this mode, and renders it objectionable. Too long walks, going out in slippery weather, dancing, hastily running up stairs, lifting heavy weights, &c., should be carefully avoided. Abortion and premature delivery are frequently the consequences of imprudence. The air she breathes should be pure; and, therefore, if possible, she ought to select a large and well ventilated bedroom. Intense anxiety about anything, severe study, and night watchings, are decidedly injurious.

DISORDERS OF PREGNANCY.

Although the state of pregnancy is perfectly natural and perfectly healthy, yet in consequence of the existence of latent diseases in some constitutions naturally, the artificial disorders produced in others by improper medical treatment, and sometimes from accidental causes, it often happens that this condition is attended by many deviations from health; which it may be well to notice, together with the best means of removing them.

Notwithstanding the universally admitted tendency to plethora, and general fullness of the system during gestation, the preposterous idea of depletion being necessary to get rid of that fullness, must not be entertained.

Hear what Dr. Dewees says on the subject of bleeding in certain cases: "To women who are in the habit of miscarrying, this proscription of indiscriminate bleeding is particularly important, especially as it is the remedy almost universally resorted to for its relief; than which, in very many instances, nothing can be more preposterous or improper. We know ourselves to be justified in saying, it has very often produced the evil it was intended to prevent." (Dewees on children, p. 28.)

The state of nervous excitation incident to pregnancy is susceptible of successful treatment; and,

Under judicious management, the storm, which sometimes seems to threaten the safety of the patient, can be so directed as to give a new impetus to the current of life, and render the woman more healthy than before.

We shall now proceed to notice some of the disturbances which take place during pregnancy, and point out the treatment of such of them as call for medicine.

VERTIGO AND HEADACHE.

Sometimes as early as the second week, but generally in the third week after conception, a strange sensation of fullness or heaviness is felt in the head, attended with dullness, and a disinclination to active employment. If these feelings increase, the sensation of lightness of the head follows, with vertigo, especially in the morning giddiness, with blindness after stooping; scintillations before the eyes; sleepiness, or its opposite headache, with weight on the head or in the back of the neck; disposition to fall forwards when stooping; palpitation of the heart; general nervousness, &c. With the above symptoms in many cases at this early period may be noticed a fastidious state of the stomach; variable, and, on the whole, diminished appetite; the smell of food while it is cooking becomes disgusting; provisions as they are exhibited in market excite nausea; articles of diet in common use, of which the patient may have been fond, becomes offensive; and articles that she could not eat before are now taken with avidity. It is remarkable that these likes and dislikes are not the result of actual experiment, but arise from a capriciousness of taste, which decides the matter before the article has been tasted at all. The tongue is occasionally coated yellow, with slightly increased redness along the middle towards the point, or the whole tongue is whitish, and enlarged. The mouth fills with tasteless saliva.

Perhaps no single case of pregnancy is attended with all the unpleasant symptoms above mentioned, a few only being present in each case, and even those may be so mild as to attract but little notice, and in some instances the woman enjoys uninterrupted health throughout the period of gestation.

Aconite, vertigo on rising from a seat, often, as if intoxicated, causing one to fall; faintness on rising from a recumbent posture, with dimness of vision; congestion of blood to the head, with throbbing and pressure in the forehead; stupefying pains in the head; eyes red and sparkling, with intolerance of light; black spots before the eyes. This remedy is chiefly applicable to plethoric persons, with a florid complexion and nervous temperament.

Dose.—Three globules dissolved in a teaspoonful of water every two or three hours, until relief is obtained.

Belladonna, vertigo, with staggering and trembling; stupor, with loss of consciousness; fullness of the head, with whizzing in the ears and danger of falling; intolerance of noise; heaviness, and pressure on the head, or in the forehead, above the eyes; expansive pains in the head, with violent beating of the carotid arteries; injected eyes—quivering of the lids, and redness of the face; sparks before the eyes; objects appear double. The symptoms requiring the use of Belladonna are generally worse in the morning, and the patient dislikes to move.

Dose.—Dissolve twelve globules in half a tumbler of water, and take a teaspoonful every one or two hours according to circumstances.

Nux vomica, vertigo, and bewildered feeling in the head; giddiness, with cloudiness of the eyes and buzzing in the ears; tearing, drawing, and jerking pains in the head; periodical pains; sufferings about the head, of almost every description, during pregnancy; accompanied with constipation, disgust of food, with insipidity, or acid, bitter, and putrid taste in the mouth. Well suited to persons of a quick, hasty disposition, and especially to such as lead sedentary lives and are addicted to the use of coffee. The sufferings are generally worse in the morning, after exercise, and on coming in from the open-air.

Dose.—Six globules every night before going to bed, and if no improvement, repeat it again in the morning.

Opium, vertigo on rising up; vertigo with stupidity, as after a debauch; imperfect sleep, with lethargy and puffed face; illusions of the imagination.

Dose.—Four globules, dry, upon the tongue, or dissolved in a teaspoonful of clear water, every three hours, until amelioration or change.

Platina, headache that increases gradually and then diminishes in the same way; headache caused by vexation or a fit of passion; spitting of tasteless or sweetish saliva; sufferings of nervous and hysterical females, which are aggravated during repose and relieved by motion.

Dose.—Four globules morning and night.

Pulsatilla, vertigo, worse after stooping, with momentary blindness, staggering and danger of falling; one-sided headache; pulsating and shooting pains in the head; sympathetic headache, arising from the stomach; headache every other day: the sufferings are frequently attended with numbness of the limbs—are generally worse in the evening and before midnight. Pulsatilla is particularly adapted to the sufferings of good-natured people, of a gentle disposision.

Dose.—Dissolve twelve globules in half a tumbler of pure water, and take a teaspoonful every two or three hours, until relief is obtained.

MORNING SICKNESS, &c.

This common, but often times very distressing concomitant of pregnancy, usually begins about six weeks after conception, and continues with more or less violence until the sixteenth week. After this time it generally abates, but in some instances it returns from slight provocations to the end of gestation. Nausea and vomiting commonly take place as soon as the patient rises from her bed, and very often continue to harrass her for two or three hours through the morning. After considerable straining and gagging, a mouthful of tough mucus is thrown up, which at times is so sour as to set the teeth on edge. There is rarely any food ejected, but occasionally bile is discharged in considerable quantities.

In this connexion may also be noticed the spitting of frothy saliva, and the more profuse salivation, which sometimes attend pregnancy. The frothy saliva, which causes the spitting, is very white and tenacious; when it falls upon the floor it assumes a circular shape, and hence the woman is said to be spitting "fippennybits." In some cases the salivation is very profuse, and attended by heartburn and waterbrash.

REMEDIES. *Arsenicum*, *Ipecacuanha*, *Natrum muriaticum*, *Nux vomica*, and *Pulsatilla*.

Arsenicum is useful, when there is excessive vomiting after eating or drinking, with attacks of fainting, great weakness, and emaciation.

Dose.—Four globules in a teaspoonful of water after each spell, or repeated at intervals of six hours, until four doses have been given, and afterwards once a day until amelioration or change.

Ipecacuanha, violent vomiting with pains in the pit of the stomach; coated tongue; vomiting of bile; vomiting, with thirst; loss of appetite, and looseness of the bowels.

Dose.—Six globules twice a day, until amelioration or change.

Natrum muriaticum, in obstinate cases, with waterbrash; clawing in the pit of the stomach, which is painful to the touch; acidity of the stomach; salivation; loss of taste and appetite.

Dose.—Four globules morning and night until improvement takes place.

Nux vomica, vomiting, with vertigo, restlessness, and ill humor; vomiting of sour mucus; bitter taste in the mouth; continual nausea; heartburn; waterbrash; hiccup; painful sensibility, with pressure in the pit of the stomach as if caused by a stone.

Dose.—Three globules in a tablespoonful of water, every night at bed-time, until improvement manifests itself; but if no improvement shows itself in forty-eight hours, consider the next remedy.

Pulsatilla, tongue coated white; insupportable

nausea, with desire to vomit; vomiting of sour mucus and food; nausea rising into the throat and mouth; eructations, acid, bitter, or with the taste of food; bitter or sour taste in the mouth after eating; nausea after eating; salivation; water-brash; hiccups; pulsations in the pit of the stomach; frequent inclination to pass water. &c.

Dose.—Six globules twice a day.

PRURITUS.

During the early months, but sometimes not until a later period of pregnancy, women are subject to a very troublesome and distressing itching of the vulva, or private parts. In almost every case of pregnancy there is an increase of the secretion of mucus of those parts, and in some instances, there is an acridity of the secretion, which gives rise to this complaint. An aphthous efflorescence, similar to the thrush of infants, occasionally incrusts the inner surfaces of the labia and adjacent parts in this disease; sometimes the affection penetrates to considerable depth in the direction of the womb. In other instances the aphthous condition is not present; but, in place of it, there is a great deal of irritation of the same parts, which assume a copper color, and present a number of slight abrasions. From the whole of the parts laboring under this peculiar irritation a vitiated watery discharge seems to be almost constantly oozing; the accumulation of which is attended with the most indomitable itching. This disease is not confined to the state of pregnancy, but may attack a female at any time; she is most liable to it, however, during gestation, and at the decline of the menses.

Frequent ablutions with water are very important for the comfort of the patient, and, at the same time, conducive to her recovery.

The principal remedies are: *Bryonia*, *Carbo vegetabilis*, *Lycopodium*, *Pulsatilla*, *Sepia*, *Silicea*, and *Magnesia muriaticum*.

Carbo vegetabilis, itching or burning; soreness of the pudendum; pain as from excoriation of the pudendum, with leucorrhœa—it is peculiarly adapted to the aphthous variety of eruptions.

Dose.—Six globules twice a day until relief is obtained.

Silicia, great irritability and sensitiveness of the skin, itching of the pudendum, with discharge of painful smarting leucorrhœa, or discharge of milky fluid, from the womb, which causes violent itching of the parts.

Dose.—Six globules twice a day, until four doses are taken, and then wait a week.

Bryonia and *Lycopodium* are applicable in case of dryness and heat in the parts.

Lycopodium is also applicable when there is a milky ichorous discharge, with or without the expulsion of wind from the parts.

Pulsatilla is suited to every variety of the disease, especially if it occur at the period of the decline of the menses.

Sepia, violent itching, with inflammation and swelling of the labia; corrosive leucorrhœa, with bearing down, and excoriation about the parts.

Dose.—The above remedies should be given the same as directed for Silicea, always selecting the remedy in accordance with the symptoms.

Magnesia muriaticum, when the irritation is attended with a thick leucorrhœal discharge, occasionally streaked with blood.

Dose.—Six globules night and morning.

A wash made of a solution of borax in water, applied locally two or three times a day, will temporarily remove the troublesome symptom of itching in a short time.

HEARTBURN AND WATERBRASH.

These affections generally go together, and may attack a woman during any part of the period of gestation. They may come on in the early months, and accompany the morning sickness, &c.; but generally they come on later in the term, and are most troublesome after quickening.

The patient complains of heat in the stomach, extending upwards; it is frequently attended with very acid eructations. There is usually a cramp-like sensation in the pit of the stomach; rising of a tasteless or bitter fluid, which is sometimes hot, and so acrid as to excoriate the throat and mouth. The symptoms are worse after eating, and water frequently turns sour, and is regurgitated immediately after drinking.

REMEDIES. *Nux vomica*, *Phosphoric acid*, *Pulsatilla*, *Sulphur*, *Calcarea carb.*, and *Alumina.*

Nux vomica, acid, bitter, or sour eructations, with nausea and vomiting; feeling of weight in the pit of the stomach; desire for chalk or earth; constipation; also when it is brought on by the too frequent use of spiritous liquors; bitter or putrid taste in the mouth, with vomiting of food in the evening.

Dose.—Dissolve twelve globules in a tumbler half full of water, and take a teaspoonful every two, three, or four hours, according to circumstances.

Phosphoric acid, sour eructations; constant nausea; dryness and soreness of the throat; eructation caused by the use of acids; vomiting of food; loss of appetite; accumulation of viscid mucus in the mouth, after taste of food, and nausea after eating.

Dose.—Four globules three times a day, until amelioration or change.

Pulsatilla, sour, bitter, bilious eructations after a meal; frequent gulping up of a bitter fluid; vomiting; eructations tasting of the food; nausea while eating, with aversion.

Dose.—Dissolve twelve globules in a tumbler half full of water, and take a teaspoonful every four hours until better.

Sulphur, sour risings, with much acidity of the stomach; nausea, with desire to vomit; sour vomiting, or vomiting of the food taken; flat, or putrid taste in the morning on rising, with complete loss of appetite, and continual thirst.

Dose.—Four globules three or four times a day, according to the violence of the case.

Calcarea carbonicum, waterbrash from taking milk; burning in the throat; bad taste in the mouth, which is metalic or sour; loss of appetite, with acidity of the stomach; aversion to food; frequent eructations after eating.

Dose.—The same as directed for Pulsatilla.

Alumina, gulping up of sour mucus, with burning in the throat; frequent eructations—bitter, rancid, burning, acrid or sour; qualmishness in the stomach; nausea, with inclination to vomit.

Dose.—Six globules every four or six hours, according to circumstances.

CONSTIPATION.

Constipation is a very frequent attendant upon pregnancy. Exercise, a diet composed chiefly of vegetables, and drinking freely of cold water, will generally relieve it. But if these are not sufficient, give *Bryonia*, *Lycopodium*, *Nux vomica*, *Pulsatilla*, *Opium*, or *Sulphur*.

Bryonia is useful where constipation occurs in warm weather, or where it arises from disordered stomach; hard, tough stool, or dry, as if burnt, with protusion of the rectum, and burning after stool, and is accompanied with determination of blood to the head.

Dose.—Six globules night and morning until relief is obtained.

Lycopodium, when there is difficulty in passing stool, with ineffectual urging and distension of the abdomen; inactivity of the rectum; small stool, followed by painful accumulation of flatulence.

Dose.—Six globules every night until decided amelioration or change.

Nux vomica, when constipation is caused by taking heavy, indigestible food; inactivity of the bowels, from sedentary habits; ineffectual urging to stool; difficult stool, with burning in the anus; constipation, with rush of blood to the head.

Dose.—Six globules night and morning until decided improvement or change.

Pulsatilla, when constipation is brought on by the too great use of rich or fat food, as pork, pastry, &c.; or there is an alternation of costive ness and diarrhœa, with painful pressing in the back.

Dose.—The same as directed for Nux vomica.

Opium, where there is constipation caused by torpor of the intestines, brought on by the abuse of cathartics; hard stool, with discharge of small, hard balls; loss of appetite; suitable for persons of a strong plethoric habit.

Dose.—Four globules night and morning until decided amelioration or change.

Sulphur is best adapted to cases of chronic constipation; especially if accompanied with piles, and the stools are hard and difficult; or lumpy, with burning pains in the anus and rectum.

Dose.—Six globules every night until relief is obtained.

DIARRHŒA.

Diarrhœa is not so common as constipation during pregnancy, but is much more injurious. It should not be suffered to continue long, lest it lead to something more serious. It frequently depends on some accidental cause, on the removal of which, the diarrhœa ceases spontaneously.

The best remedies are: *Antimonium crudum*, *Dulcamara*, *Lycopodium*, *Sulphur*, and *Phosphorus*.

Antimonium crudum, where there is a disposition to diarrhœa, or diarrhœa from taking cold; diarrhœa at night, with discharge of mucus from the rectum, which is protruded during stool; or when the diarrhœa is alternate with constipation, or if the discharges are watery and very offensive.

Dose.—Four globules every three hours until relief is obtained.

Dulcamara will promptly afford relief if the attack has been brought on by sudden suppression of perspiration or chill, and the discharges are slimy, or sour smelling, with colic, especially in the summer season.

Dose.—Six globules every two hours until amelioration or change.

Lycopodium, diarrhœa with colic; pale, fetid stools, with burning; stools followed by spasms of the abdomen; hæmorrhage from the rectum, with soft stools; cutting in the rectum.

Dose.—Six globules every four hours until amelioration or change.

Sulphur, diarrhœa after a cold, with chilliness, colic, and distension of the abdomen; discharges brown, green, or watery; fetid or sour smelling stools; burning during stool; discharge of undigested food with stool.

Dose.—Six globules three times a day until relief is obtained, or the symptoms indicate another remedy.

Phosphorus is suitable in obstinate cases, where the discharges are painless, involuntary, and watery, soft and pupescent, or green, black, and undigested.

Dose.—Four globules every four hours until relief is obtained.

TOOTHACHE.

Toothache is most common in the early months of pregnancy, and is sometimes one of its first symptoms. It is liable to occur at any time during the term, and usually comes on in paroxysms after longer or shorter intervals. It may attack one or more decayed teeth, or a perfectly sound tooth; or shoot along the jaw without locating in any particular tooth. The pain partakes of the nature of neuralgia. Consult a physician before having teeth extracted under such circumstances.

The most successful remedies are: *Aconite*, *Belladonna*, *Calcarea carb.*, *Chammomilla*, *Nux vomica*, *Pulsatilla*, and *Staphysagria*.

Aconite, in congestive toothache, if there is intense redness of the cheek; congestion of the head; great restlessness, and throbbing pain in the face, with burning heat; and is aggravated by all kinds of stimulants.

Dose.—Six globules every hour until amelioration or change.

Belladonna, tearing or cutting pain in the gums

and teeth, as if ulcerated; worse at night, especially after lying down; face hot and red; worse from the contact of food, or in the open air; cheeks swollen; dryness of the mouth and throat, with great thirst; burning and redness of the eyes.

Dose.—Six globules every two or three hours according to circumstances.

Calcarea carbonica, toothache, with congestion of blood to the head; worse at night, with beating pain or soreness; aggravated by anything warm or cold, and by the least noise.

Dose.—Six globules dissolved in three tablespoonfuls of water, and a teaspoonful every hour until relief is obtained.

Chammomilla, violent drawing or beating pains, which appear intolerable, especially at night; irritable mood, with hot swelling of the cheeks; painful swelling of the gums, aggravated by the use of coffee; pains, with heat and redness, especially of one side of the face; restlessness and great weakness.

Dose.—Four globules every one or two hours until relief is obtained.

Nux vomica, applicable to those who lead a sedentary life, or of a lively, choleric temperament; the pains extend to the head and ears; aggravated by the use of spiritous drinks; better in the air; swelling of the glands of the neck; renewal of the pains at night; swelling and sensitiveness of the gums.

Dose.—The same as directed for Chammomilla.

Pulsatilla, applicable to persons of a mild, quiet, and timid disposition; where the pains extend to the ears, and wander from one side to the other, with jerking pains, as if the nerves were put upon the stretch and suddenly loosed again; face pale; heat in the head, with chilliness of the body, aggravated by any thing warm; relieved by the use of cold water and fresh air.

Dose.—Four globules every one, two, or three hours, as circumstances may require.

Staphysagria, gums painful, pale, ulcerated, and swollen, bleeding easily; pain in all the teeth; pains worse when chewing, or after drinking anything cold.

Dose.—The same as of Pulsatilla.

PENDULOUS ABDOMEN.

Females who have borne many children are liable to this deformity of the abdomen, especially where there is a disposition to corpulency, and where proper attention has not been paid to the *bandage* in previous confinements.

REMEDIES. *Rhus toxicodendron* and *Sepia*.

Rhus toxicodendron, where there is considerable

relaxation of the abdominal muscles during pregnancy, and also after confinement.

Dose.—Six globules every night

Sepia will be found useful, especially where there is a tendency to this affection, with a sense of weight in the abdomen.

Dose.—Six globules every night.

VARICOSE VEINS.

This disease consists of a dilatation and distension of the veins. It is not confined to a state of pregnancy, but may exist at any time in the female, and occasionally is met with in the male sex. Still the disease is so frequently met with in women during pregnancy, that it may be considered as a disease almost peculiar to this state. It rarely occurs in a first pregnancy; and when it appears for the first time, it does not commonly occur until after the period of quickening; but in subsequent pregnancies it is apt to take place in the early months.

Varicose veins generally appear first about the ankle, and are frequently confined to the leg below the knee; but occasionally the veins of the entire lower extremity are involved. The affection may be confined to one limb, or both may be included. Oedema, or general swelling of the feet or lower limbs, may attend this complaint or exist without it.

The enlarged veins are generally superficial, and at first assume a reddish hue, but afterwards a bluish or leaden color, and the larger ones become very much knotted; they get larger when the patient stands on her feet, or suffers the limb to hang down, and the swelling decreases when she lies down.

When moderate it is not painful, but if it continues to increase it may become so, and ultimately the veins may burst, and the blood be effused beneath the skin, or poured out externally. As the disease is produced by a mechanical cause, after delivery, the pressure being removed, the veins very soon regain their natural size and the swelling disappears.

If the distension is great, and the disease be very painful, rest in the recumbent posture will be necessary. If the woman is obliged to be on her feet much, she will find great relief from having the limb bandaged, or wearing the laced stocking. If the bandage or laced stocking is used, it should be applied in the morning, when the veins are least distended, beginning at the toes and progressing upwards.

In addition to the above mechanical means the following medicines may be given with advantage, namely: *Aconite*, *Lycopodium*, *Nux vomica*, and *Pulsatilla.*

Aconite, heaviness in the limbs, with lameness of the joints, as if they were bruised; lacerating pain in the muscles of the legs; standing becomes painful; all the pains increase by standing or moving about.

Dose.—Twelve globules dissolved in a tumbler half full of water, and take a teasponful every four hours.

Lycopodium, drawing pain in the limbs, as if bruised, with tension and stiffness; large, red, hot patches, painful and burning, extending from the knees to the ancles; worse at night, with heat and dryness of the skin.

Dose.—Six globules dissolved in a teaspoonful of water, night and morning.

Nux vomica, weariness and unsteadines of the limbs; coldness, with frequent dartings from the feet to the thighs; painful tension in the muscles, as if too short; blue spots in the legs, as if ecchymosed, with tensive pain; or if there is constipation or hemorrhoids.

Dose.—Six globules in a teaspoonful of water, morning, noon, and night.

Pulsatilla, if the swelling is red and hot, with excessive pain and inflammation; unsteadiness and weakness in the knees, with blueness of the entire veins of the legs, extending from the knees to the ankles.

Dose.—Four globules three times a day, either dry on the tongue, or dissolved in a little water.

HEMORRHOIDS OR PILES.

Although this disease is not by any means peculiar to pregnancy alone, yet it often arises in persons while in this state who are not subject to it at any other time, from the pressure of the gravid uterus and a torpid condition of the abdominal viscera.

Piles consist of one or more small vascular tumors about the anus. When severe, they enlarge to the size of marbles, and form a cluster like a compact bunch of grapes, of a purplish hue, and are very painful and sensitive to the touch. When they occupy the lower part of the rectum within the anus, they are called inward piles; and when they protrude, they are called external piles. If there is no discharge from them, they are called blind piles; and when there is a discharge from them, they are called bleeding piles.

A patient, who is liable to piles, or somewhat afflicted with them, should neither sit too much, nor stand on her feet long at a time, but take plenty of exercise, drink freely of cold water, and abstain from all rich food and stimulating drinks.

During a paroxysm of suffering from them, it will be expedient for her to lie down, and choose for herself the easiest position. As a local application, place a folded napkin wet in cold water next to them, and lay a dry one folded in like manner over it, and repeat the process as occasion may require. Any animal oil, or a mucilage made by soaking quince-seeds in water, and applied, will frequently give temporary relief; but for more permanent benefit, we must resort to one or more of the following medicines, according to the symptoms, namely: *Aconite*, *Belladonna*, *Ignatia*, *Nux vomica*, and *Sulphur*.

Aconite is applicable when there is bleeding, with cutting or pricking pains, and pressure at the anus; fullness in the abdomen, with tightness and colic; and pain in the small of the back, as if it was broken.

Dose.—Six globules dissolved in a wineglassful of water, and a teaspoonful three times a day until relief is obtained, or the symptoms indicate another remedy.

Belladonna, when the bleeding continues for several days, with itching of the anus, and soreness when walking; tumors large, with bearing down; pain in the back, as if it would break. Belladonna is especially indicated if the patient have taken sulphur in large doses, under old school treatment in previous attacks.

Dose.—The same as directed for Aconite.

Ignatia, constipation, with ineffectual efforts at stool; body comes down; protrusion of the piles during a laxative evacuation, with discharge of bloody mucus; painful pressure after stool; contractive feeling in the anus; itching and crawling in the anus.

Dose.—Six globules night and morning, until amelioration or change manifests itself, or another remedy should be required.

Nux vomica is applicable for both blind and bleeding piles, attended by constipation, and frequent ineffectual efforts at stool, with a sensation as if the anus were contracted or closed; burning and pricking pain in the tumors; itching in the anus; colicky pains in the abdomen; determination to the head; frequent painful urination; worse after mental labor and after a meal. Particularly adapted to persons of sedentary habits, and who use much coffee.

Dose.—Four globules dissolved in a teaspoonful of water, night and morning.

Sulphur, when there is alternate constipation and diarrhœa; sensation of excoriation, with itching and burning at the anus; frequent protrusion of the tumors; fullness of the head; sour stomach; dyspepsia; painful urination; morning diarrhœa, with bearing down and protrusion of the rectum. In obstinate cases, give Nux vomica and Sulphur alternately, night and morning.

Dose.—Six globules night and morning.

PAIN IN THE RIGHT SIDE.

After the fifth month of pregnancy, some women are attacked with a deep-seated pain in the right side under the ribs. The sensation is that of constant aching, attended with heat. The patient cannot sit long at a time. The pain gets easier after being in bed for an hour or two at night. It generally leaves at the beginning of the eighth month. Short women, particularly in their first pregnancies, are most likely to suffer from this complaint.

REMEDIES. *Aconite*, *Chamomilla*, and *Pulsatilla*.

Aconite, drawing pain in the side, extending to the navel, aggravated by stooping; pressure in the region of the liver, which is very sensitive to the touch, with oppression and arrest of breathing.

Dose.—Three globules every four hours, until relief is manifest.

Chamomilla, aching pain under the ribs, causing oppressed breathing, especially after taking coffee; abdomen hard and distended.

Dose.—Disssolve twelve globules in three tablespoonfuls of water, and take a teaspoonful every two hours.

Pulsatilla, sticking pain in the region of the

liver, especially when walking; spasms and lacerating pain in the abdomen of pregnant females; increase of pain in the side during pregnancy.

Dose.—The same as directed for Chamomilla.

CRAMPS.

This very annoying affection is mostly worse about the fourth and fifth months, and again towards the end of pregnancy.

Cramps may attack the muscles of the abdomen, the back, the hips, and the lower extremities.

For cramps in the muscles of the abdomen, take *Belladonna*, *Hyoscyamus*, *Nux vomica*, or *Pulsatilla*.

When they attack the back, take *Ignatia*, *Opium*, or *Rhus toxicodendron*.

Hips, *Colocynth*, *Graphites*, or *Stramonium*.

Thighs, *Hyoscyamus*.

Legs, *Calcarea carbonica*, *Chamomilla*, *Nux vomica*, if after midnight, or *Sulphur*, if in the evening.

Feet, *Calcarea carbonica*.

Dose.—Dissolve twelve globules in a wine-glass of water, and take of the solution a teaspoonful every half, one, two, or three hours, according to circumstances.

INCONTINENCE OF URINE.

This very distressing complaint may occur at any time during pregnancy, but perhaps is most common during the early months. If the inclination is not attended to immediately, the urine is discharged involuntarily. The urine is frequently very acrid, and possessed of a strong odor.

REMEDIES. *Belladonna*, *Cina*, *Pulsatilla*, *Silicea*, and *Stramonium*.

Belladonna, frequent and copious emission of urine, especially at night; inability to retain the urine from relaxation of the neck of the bladder, without desire to urinate; urine pale and watery, or yellow and turbid.

Dose.—Four globules every six hours, until relief is obtained.

Cina, frequent desire to urinate, with copious emission; also, involuntary emission of urine at night.

Dose.—The same as directed for Belladonna.

Pulsatilla, frequent desire to urinate, with drawing in the abdomen; spasmodic pain in the neck of the bladder; urine watery and colorless.

Dose.—Six globules three times a day.

Silicea, desire to urinate, with smarting in the urethra, and copious emission.

Dose.—Six globules every night, until four doses are taken.

Stramonium, urine profuse, with involuntary emission.

Dose.—Six globules three times a day.

PAINFUL URINATION.

This concomitant of pregnancy is relieved by *Cocculus*, *Phosphoric acid*, *Pulsatilla*, *Nux vomica*, or *Sulphur*.

Cocculus, desire to urinate, with scanty emission, and pains in the urethra.

Dose.—Four globules three times a day.

Phosphoric acid, desire to urinate, with burning pain and scanty emission; anguish and uneasiness before micturition.

Dose.—The same as Cocculus.

Pulsatilla, ineffectual urging to urinate, with difficult emission, and drawing in the abdomen; after urinating, pain in the neck of the bladder.

Dose.—Twelve globules dissolved in half a tumblerful of water, and a teaspoonful every two or three hours.

Nux vomica, painful ineffectual desire to urinate, with discharge drop by drop; burning and lacerating pain in the neck of the bladder.

Dose.—The same as directed for Pulsatilla.

Sulphur, violent desire to urinate, with discharge by drops; requiring great efforts to pass urine.

Dose.—The same as directed for Pulsatilla.

SLEEPLESSNESS.

Towards the latter end of pregnancy, many women, to use their own expression, become so fidgety at night, that they cannot sleep. This condition is often attended with sleepiness; but just as sleep is approaching, the limbs jerk, or restlessness suddenly comes over the patient, and she is obliged to move, which dissipates for a little time the disposition to sleep. Some can sleep well enough in the daytime.

Air and exercise, not carried to the extent of producing fatigue, are the best preventatives.

Belladonna, *Coffea*, *Hyoscyamus*, *Lycopodium*, *Nux vomica*, and *Opium*, are the best remedies.

Belladonna, sleeplessness at night, with drowsiness, restlessness, and tossing about; starting as in a fright, especially when on the point of falling asleep; frequent waking, with difficulty of going to sleep again.

Dose.—Six globules dissolved in a tablespoonful of water, before going to bed.

Coffea, restless sleep the whole night; weariness; nervousness; waking, with starting, owing to agitation of body and mind.

Dose.—Dissolve twelve globules in a tumbler half full of water, and take a teaspoonful every two, three, or four hours, according to circumstances.

Hyoscyamus, sleeplessness from nervous irritation; or, as if caused by fright, starting from sleep.

Dose.—The same as directed for Coffea.

Lycopodium, drowsiness; restless sleep; light sleep, full of fancies; starting in the sleep, with jerking of the limbs.

Dose.—Six globules dissolved in a tablespoonful of water, to be taken before going to bed.

Nux vomica, constant disposition to sleep; drowsiness after meal; light sleep at night, with frequent waking; violent starting on going to sleep.

Dose.—The same as directed for Coffea.

Opium, drowsiness, with great inclination to sleep; starting in the sleep, with jerking in the limbs; restless sleep, with moaning and groaning; or sleep full of dreams.

Dose.—Six globules dissolved in a tablespoonful of water, night and morning.

MELANCHOLY.

Under this head may also be included, *Despondency*, *Hypocondriasis*, *Lowness of Spirits*, *&c.* It is not my intention here to enter upon a long detail of symptoms, but I would make a lump job of it by saying, that the unfortunate subject of this unhappy state of mind always looks on the dark side of the picture, and sees everything through an unfavorable medium. She seems to realize in her own feelings every unpropitious symptom she ever heard of, and is even afraid that something still worse awaits her. Gossips and injudicious friends frequently unwittingly contribute to this morbid state of feeling, by relating an account of accidents and unhappy issues which perhaps never occurred.

Aconite, if the fear of death be predominant, and if the unhappy state of mind have been caused by fright.

Dose.—Three globules dissolved in a teaspoonful of water, three times a day until relief is obtained.

Aurum, melancholy, with desire for death; irresistible desire to weep; anguish of mind which prompts one to commit suicide; despondency; weakness of the memory and intellectual faculties.

Dose.—Six globules dissolved in half a tumbler of water, and a tablespoonful to be taken every three or four hours.

Belladonna, great agitation and inquietude at night; fearfulness, with inclination to run away, or hide; fear of ghosts; involuntary laughter; disposition to laugh and sing, or to become furious with rage; dread of exertion; illusions of the senses; frightful visions, &c.

Dose.—The same as prescribed for Aconite.

Pulsatilla, sadness and tears; oppressed with a multitude of cares; distress in the pit of the stomach; sleeplessness, headache, and heartburn; she sits in a taciturn mood, folds her hands upon her lap, and says foolish things; moroseness, with repugnancy to conversation.

Dose.—Four globules three times a day.

Sulphur, depression of spirits, with great concern on the subject of religion; despair of salvation; forgetfulness of proper names, and especially of words when about to speak them; disposition to get angry.

Dose.—Six globules dissolved in a tablespoonful of water, night and morning.

FAINTING AND HYSTERIC FITS.

These affections may take place at any time during the period of gestation, but they are most apt to occur about the time of quickening. Robust women may have them, but such attacks are generally confined to the nervous and delicate. The patient first feels a sensation of languor, with inclination to yawn; everything appears to turn round; her sight becomes obscure; buzzing and ringing in the ears; her face turns pale; she sighs and becomes insensible. There are no convulsive motions, no choking with noise in the throat, and no biting of the tongue as in epileptic fits.

They may be caused by fright, anger, and alarm of any kind, and sometimes they occur without any external exciting cause.

Aconite, *Chamomilla*, or *Ignatia*, if they are caused by a fit of passion or fright.

Dose.—Dissolve six globules in a wineglassful of water, and give a teaspoonful every ten or fifteen minutes, according to circumstances.

Belladonna, when there is determination of blood to the head, with flushed face; heat of the head, with coldness of the extremities.

Dose.—The same as above directed for Aconite.

Ignatia, when there is severe headache; nausea and fainting; chilliness, with paleness of the face; the patient can bear neither light nor noise; distension of the abdomen.

Dose.—If the spells are protracted, or recur repeatedly, dissolve twelve globules in three tablespoonfuls of water, and give a teaspoonful every five, ten, or fifteen minutes until relief is obtained.

Pulsatilla, when there is a disposition to shed tears, and in persons of great nervous susceptibility.

Dose.—The same as directed for Belladonna.

MISCARRIAGE AND FLOODING.

On account of the very intimate association of

these two diseases of pregnancy, I have concluded to give their treatment conjointly. If they were treated of separately, there would be frequent repetition of the same symptoms.

Abortion may frequently be prevented even after flooding and labor pains have commenced; and, in cases where this cannot be done, the sufferings of the patient may be very much mitigated, and the evil consequences partially avoided. It may occur at any period of gestation, but is most frequent at the third month. If it occurs after the sixth month, it is called premature labor. It may result from accidental causes, constitutional predisposition, or some latent disease.

Arnica, if it is caused by a blow; lifting heavy weights; overreaching; a fall; or any other violent concussion; when pains, which bear down heavily, or real labor pains make their appearance, with a mixed discharge from the vagina.

Dose.—Twelve globules dissolved in half a glass of water, and a teaspoonful to be given every half, one, or two hours; or, if the case is very urgent, it may be repeated every ten or fifteen minutes until amelioration or change.

Belladonna, when there are violent pressing pains, with tension in the whole abdomen, particularly low down, with the feeling as if the private parts would fall out, which is characteristic for Belladonna; pain in the small of the back, as if it would break; the patient is pale and restless, or her face is flushed, and she is stupid; heat about the head; thirst; palpitation; the discharge is neither very dark, nor very bright red.

Dose.—The same as directed for Arnica.

Bryonia, the discharge is of a dark color, in large quantities, with pain in the small of the back; headache, particularly in the temples, as if the head would burst; especially if constipation attend.

Dose.—Three globules dissolved in a teaspoonful of water every one, two, or three hours, according to circumstances.

Chamomilla, when there are violent pains going from the back around the stomach, resembling an inclination to evacuate the bowels, or pass water; the pains are periodical, like labor pains, and each one is followed by a dark and coagulated discharge; much thirst; and coldness of the extremities.

Dose.—The same as directed for Bryonia.

China is very important in the most dangerous cases of flooding; when heaviness of the head, giddiness, loss of consciousness, and drowsiness appear; sudden weakness; coldness of the extremities; fainting; paleness of the face; convulsions of the mouth; contortions of the eyes; the face and hands turn blue; single jerks pass through the whole body; the discharge passes by starts, and may be either thin and bright red, or dark and coagulated; the cramp-like contraction is attended with a painful sensation of bearing down towards the anus, and the discharge is increased at every pain. During the administration of this remedy, cloths dipped in vinegar and water may be applied to the lower part of the stomach. Afterwards a little wine and water may be given. China always answers well for the debility, and other troublesome symptoms which sometimes remain after the flooding has ceased. Should there be colicky pains, with frequent inclination to pass water, and sore tension of the abdomen afterwards, give Aconite.

Dose.—The same as directed for Arnica.

Hyoscyamus, when there are spasmodic affections of the whole body, or jerking of single limbs, sometimes caused by stiffness of the joints and loss of consciousness, attended with a light red discharge, which is worse during the spasms and at night. The pains resemble labor pains, with drawing in the thighs, and small of the back; heat over the whole body, with quick, full pulse, with fullness of the veins on the back of the hands and in the face; great uneasiness; excessive liveliness; trembling over the whole body; numbness of the limbs; darkness before the eyes; delirium, and twitching of the sinews of the wrists.

Dose.—Dissolve twelve globules in a wineglassful of water, and give a teaspoonful every one, two, or three hours, according to the severity of the symptoms.

Ipecacuanha, when the threatened miscarriage is attended with spasmodic affections, without loss of consciousness; copious flooding; the discharge flows without interruption, but is worse during motion, with cutting pains around the navel, and great pressure downwards; chills, and coldness of the body; internal heat rising towards the head; great weakness, and inclination to lie down.

Dose.—The same as directed for Bryonia.

Nux vomica, threatened abortion, particularly about the third month; spasmodic pains, accompanied with ineffectual urging to stool; the pains are accompanied with nausea, and sometimes faintness; strong bearing down, with frequent inclination to pass water, and heat in the private parts; discharge of mucus.

Dose.—The same as directed for Hyoscyamus.

Platina, when the discharge is dark, thick, and sometimes coagulated; the pain in the back draws towards the groins, with pressing down internally to the private parts, which are excessively sensitive. Particularly applicable where mental emotions are the cause.

Dose.—The same as directed for Bryonia.

Administration. On the first appearance of the premonitory symptoms of miscarriage, the patient should keep quiet or go to bed, release her mind from care, avoid exciting conversation, and live on a light diet. Select the remedy according to the symptoms, and if better in a few hours, or the next day, repeat it as often as it becomes necessary But if no improvement follow in a short time, select another remedy. If better, take nothing more so long as the improvement continues; if the symptoms return, repeat the last remedy once more before selecting another. If the symptoms are urgent, or the flooding severe, dissolve about ten pellets in a wineglassful of water, and take a teaspoonful every half hour, or not so often, according to the necessity of the case, increasing the interval as the symptoms improve, and discontinue the medicine when the flooding ceases.

BREASTS.

A great deal of suffering from sore breasts after delivery, may be saved by paying a little attention to them, for a few months previous to confinement. Women are most liable to suffer in this way with first children. During the progress of gestation, especially with first children, and in quite young women, the breasts increase very much in size, the areolæ assume a darker color, and the nipples become enlarged, and project more than they had done previously. This change in the size and condition of the nipples is often attended with some pain, and a great deal of tenderness. Excoriation, inflammation, cracks, branny exfoliations, and very minute abscesses around them, are the most common diseases to which the nipples are liable during pregnancy.

For two or three months in the latter part of pregnancy, the whole breasts should be well bathed with cold water every morning, and rendered perfectly dry afterwards, with crass towels. For simple excoriation, or tenderness of the nipples, they may be washed two or three times a day with water, containing a few drops of the tincture of Arnica, or with brandy. In some instances a little tincture of the myrrh may be added to the brandy with advantage. For the other diseases of the nipples above mentioned, the following medicines should be administered internally, according to the indications.

REMEDIES. *Chamomilla*, *Sulphur*, *Silicea*, *Graphites*, *Belladonna*, and *Mercurius vivus*.

Chamomilla, if the nipples be highly inflamed, and ache like toothache.

Dose.—Four globules dissolved in a teaspoonful of water, three or four times a day.

Sulphur, for burning, itching, swelling, cracks, branny eruption, and the minute abscesses or pimples around the nipples.

Dose.—Twelve globules dissolved in a wineglassful of water, and a teaspoonful of the solution three times a day.

Silicea, if ulceration has taken place, and there are symptoms of hectic fever present.

Dose.—The same as directed for Sulphur.

Belladonna, if the breasts are hard and swollen, with shooting or tearing pains, and of an erysipelatous redness, which diverges from a central point like rays.

Dose.—The same as directed for Chamomilla.

Mercurius vivus, after Belladonna, if the erysipelatous inflammation should not be checked, and the breasts remain hard and painful.

Dose.—The same as of Belladonna.

REMEDIES IMMEDIATELY BEFORE LABOR.

Aconite may be given if there is much vascular excitement or fever, with hot and dry skin.

Dose.—Four globules every two hours until amelioration takes place.

Belladonna, where there is a redness of the face,

pulsation of the arteries of the head, and a congestive state of the brain.

Dose.—The same as given for Aconite.

REMEDIES most valuable in tedious and complicated labors: *Coffea*, *Aconite*, *Chamomilla*, *Belladonna*, *Nux vomica*, *Pulsatilla*, and *Sepia*.

Coffea will be found of great service where there is great restlessness, or where the pains are very violent, and occur in rapid succession.

Dose.—Six globules every ten, fifteen, or twenty minutes, as the case may require.

Aconite may be used if the patient has been addicted to the use of coffee, or it may be used in alternation with Chamomilla.

Dose.—Four globules every hour until relieved.

Belladonna will be useful where labor is protracted beyond the usual time, owing to rigidity of the parts, or where there is no disposition in the parts to relax, and when the pains are insufficient.

Dose.—The same as prescribed for Coffea.

LABOR.

The process of giving birth to a child is called labor. The average duration of gestation is thirty-nine weeks. There are three cardinal points, from which, if they occur at the usual time and in regular succession, a correct "reckoning" may be kept, and the time of labor fixed with considerable certainty.

1. The time of the last period of menstruation.

2. The commencement of morning sickness—six weeks after conception.

3. Quickening at half way—one hundred and thirty-five days from quickening to labor. Moreover, the stomach gets lower after the eighth month, and the woman is smaller around the waist the last month of her pregnancy, than she had been for six weeks previously.

Labor is ushered in by a few premonitory signs. One very common and very good one is looseness of the bowels, sometimes for a day or two before. Various nervous symptoms, such as agitation without cause, disposition to shed tears without distress, in other instances lowness of spirits, occasionally precede labor. Flying pains through the stomach, with frequent inclination to pass water, and finally, a discharge of mucus tinged with red, technically called "a show," takes place. Then come pains at intervals of longer or shorter duration, and frequently rigors or trembling without coldness.

Were it not for the acquired habits of civilized life, the process of child-bearing would be divested of much of the suffering and danger which now so commonly attend it, as almost to lead us to consider them natural concomitants. It is almost unattended with pain among savages. It would not be wise, neither is it necessary to return to savage life in order to get rid of the ills of child-bearing; but let the women in civilized life pay more attention to the natural means, both moral and physical, of developing their whole being—live more usefully and less artificially, than they now do, in deforming themselves in order to make what they call a "fine figure," and in a few generations, many of the difficulties which now exist will have disappeared.

It is not intended here to go into a minute description of the process of labor, nor to give any specific directions for its management, as I cannot suppose that any sensible person, who is not qualified, would have the temerity to undertake the care of a case, unless placed under very peculiar circumstances. Some of the deviations from the natural course, however, may be noticed, with their appropriate treatment.

INEFFECTUAL PAINS.

Chamomilla, when there is over-excitement, and excessive sensibility to pain; and anguish, and discouragement, with tossing about.

Dose.—Twelve globules dissolved in half a tumblerful of water, and a teaspoonful of the solution every fifteen, twenty, or thirty minutes, according to the circumstances of the case.

Coffea, if the pains are excessively violent, with great mental and general nervous excitement, and over sensitiveness.

Dose.—Three globules every half, one, or two hours, to allay the nervous excitement.

Nux vomica, when the pains are irregular, and the labor does not seem to progress; drawing in the back and thighs, with pressure downward, and constant inclination to evacuate the bowels and to pass water.

Dose.—The same as prescribed of Chamomilla.

Opium is especially suitable in women of a full habit, if the pains suddenly cease, and determination to the head, with redness and fullness of the face, with a state of stupor, take place.

Dose.—Three globules dissolved in a teaspoonful of water every half, or every hour, as the case may require.

Pulsatilla, if the pains are too weak, and too far apart, or, if they become weaker, as from inactivity of the womb.

Dose.—Six globules dissolved in a wineglassful of water, and give a teaspoonful every half, or one hour, according to the circumstances of the case.

TREATMENT AFTER DELIVERY.

A patient should not be disturbed immediately

after delivery, except so far as is absolutely necessary in the application of the bandage, and to render her situation as comfortable, otherwise, as circumstances will admit of. She should be allowed to rest for an hour or two, and then if no unfavorable symptoms be present to forbid it, she may be "put to bed." If she complain of general soreness, from violent, or long continued exertion, give her two doses of Arnica, internally, three or four hours apart, or, if that should not be sufficient, give Rhus in the same way. If she complain of much soreness or pain, locally, Arnica may be applied externally, in the form of lotion, prepared by mixing twenty drops of the tincture in a tumblerful of water.

Coffea, if she cannot sleep from nervous excitement, with restlessness and tossing about.

Dose.—Three globules dissolved in a teaspoonful of water every hour, until sleep is obtained.

WEAKNESS AFTER DELIVERY.

Weakness after delivery may be caused by the loss of fluids, prostration of the nervous system, or exhaustion from protracted labors.

REMEDIES. *China*, *Aconite*, *Coffea*, and *Veratrum*.

China is particularly indicated when the weakness arises from loss of blood, and is attended with sensitiveness of the nervous system, sallow countenance, and predisposition to dropsy.

Dose.—Six globules every four hours.

Aconite, where there is nervous weakness, with restlessness and want of sleep; it may be followed by Coffea, if necessary.

Dose.—Four globules every two or three hours.

Veratrum, where the restlessness is accompanied with great prostration of strength, faintness from motion, &c.

Dose.—The same as given for China.

REMEDIES which may be required soon after delivery: *Nux vomica*, *Chamomilla*, *Dulcamara*, *Bryonia*, *Sulphur*, and *Sambucus*.

Nux vomica, prostration followed by a dry heat or chilliness, then again sweat.

Dose.—Six globules every two hours.

Dulcamara, where there is sudden suppression of perspiration brought on by exposure to a draught of air, or a sudden chill.

Dose.—Six globules every two hours.

Chamomilla may be used, if there should be colic, with a relaxed state of the bowels, with great excitability and restlessness.

Dose.—Twelve globules dissolved in half a tumbler of water, and and a teaspoonful given every hour.

Bryonia, profuse perspiration, with red face; or

moist and clammy skin, with severe headache; sleeplessness, with tossing about; flashes of heat, and suppression of the lochia.

Dose.—Six globules every hour.

Sulphur may be used in similar cases, or where Bryonia has not afforded entire relief.

Dose.—The same as Bryonia.

Sambucus, excessive perspiration, brought on by keeping the room too warm, or from the use of stimulating drinks.

Dose.—Six globules every hour.

FLOODING AFTER DELIVERY.

Belladonna, when the flooding is attended with violent pressure downwards in the internal organs, as if they would be forced out, and pain in the small of the back.

Dose.—Four globules dissolved in a teaspoonful of water every half hour, until relief is obtained.

Chamomilla, if the discharge take place at intervals, with pains running round the abdomen; constant thirst; paleness of the face, and coldness of the extremities.

Dose.—The same as directed for Belladonna.

China, when the same symptoms exist as are enumerated under Chamomilla, and, in addition thereto, vertigo, dullness of the senses, desire for fresh air, and fainting. This remedy is also suitable for the debility and want of energy, after the flooding has ceased.

Dose.—Dissolve twelve globules in a tumbler half full of water, and give a teaspoonful every half, one, two, or three hours, as the circumstances of the case may require.

Ipecacuanha, when the discharge is bright red, and constant, with cutting pains in the middle of the abdomen; bearing down; nausea, with great prostration of strength, and a desire to be fanned.

Dose.—The same as directed for Belladonna.

PUERPERAL CONVULSIONS.

Diagnosis, this disease generally comes on suddenly, about five days after delivery, with violent pain in the abdomen, great distension and sensitiveness, so that the patient cannot bear the slightest touch, not even the weight of the bedclothes; pulse much accelerated; great thirst; lowness of spirits, with vomiting; urgent desire for stool, and suppression of the secretions, &c.

TREATMENT. *Cuprum*, *Chamomilla*, *Belladonna*, *Hyoscyamus*, *Stramonium*, *Ignatia*, *Ipecacuanha*, and *Cicuta*.

Cuprum, convulsive movements and distortions of the limbs, with rigidity and bending backwards; vomiting, with pains in the abdomen; loss of consciousness; blueness of the countenance;

frothing at the mouth; biting of the tongue, or clenching of the jaws, with jerking and twitching of the extremities. The paroxysms frequently come on during sleep.

Dose.—Dissolve twelve globules in six teaspoonfuls of water, and give a teaspoonful every ten minutes.

Chamomilla, for spasms characterized by convulsions of the extremites; acute pain of a cutting character in the lumbar region; distended abdomen, red, bloated face; great sensibility of the nervous system.

Dose.—Eight globules may be dissolved in a few teaspoonfuls of water, and a teasponful given at intervals of ten, fifteen, or twenty minutes, according to the urgency of the symptoms.

Belladonna, convulsive movement of the facial muscles; congestion of blood to the head, with restless tossing about; dark red, hot, and bloated face; or pale, cold face, with shuddering between the paroxysms; ineffectual bearing down; or the spasms excited by the least touch, or contradiction.

Dose.—Four globules every fifteen or thirty minutes, according to circumstances.

Hyoscyamus, when the spasms are more severe; bluish color and bloatedness of the face; loss of consciousness; oppression of the chest; involuntary emission of urine, with stertorous breathing, or clenching of the thumbs.

Dose.—The same as given of Belladonna.

Stramonium, convulsions of a similar character, with frightful visions; laughter; lamentations; convulsive movements of the extremities; pale, worn-out appearance.

Dose.—Six globules every ten, twenty, or thirty minutes, according to circumstances.

Ignatia, loss of consciousness, with involuntary screams of laughter; and jerking of the limbs, with frequent yawning and sopor.

Dose.—The same as Belladonna.

Ipecacuanha, spasmodic convulsions, with constant desire to vomit; and thirst, with pale, bloated face.

Dose.—Six globules every half hour.

Cocculus, spasms brought on by some external injury.

Dose.—Same as for Ipecacuanha.

Cicuta, convulsions, with distortions of the extremities, with pale, or yellowish complexion.

Dose.—Six globules every fifteen or thirty minutes, according to circumstances.

AFTER PAINS

After pains rarely occur with first children, and generally, they are but slight until the third or fourth. Some women never have them of any account, and others have them severely in every confinement. Something may be done towards preventing them, by patience and a little judicious management on the part of the practitioner during labor. But frequently they occur after the most skillful management.

Arnica, if a sensation of soreness accompanies the pains, with pressure on the bladder, and retention of urine.

Dose.—Six globules every hour, or two hours.

Belladonna, for the kind of bearing down so characteristic for Belladonna, and so often mentioned, with fullness about the head, and strong inclination without the ability to sleep; also, tenderness and fullness of the abdomen.

Dose.—Twelve globules dissolved in a little water, and a teaspoonful of the solution may be given every one or two hours, as the case may require.

Chamomilla or *Coffea*, if nervous excitement, with restlessness and tossing about, prevail.

Dose.—The same as directed for Belladonna.

Nux vomica, when the pains are aching, and more of the colicky kind, with violent contractions of the womb, and sometimes followed by nausea. This remedy is always suitable for excitable and hasty persons.

Dose.—Three globules dissolved in a teaspoonful of water, every one or two hours.

Pulsatilla, in persons of a mild temperament; severe, colicky pains, extending to the back; desire to vomit; sour taste; bearing down; nervousness, with disposition to shed tears. In severe cases, Nux vomica and Pulsatilla may be given alternately in water, with very good effect.

Dose.—The same as directed for Nux vomica.

Pulsatilla is very important, when the placenta is retained too long.

FALLING OFF OF THE HAIR.

Falling off of the hair of the head is another disease to which females of a delicate constitution are liable after confinement, and throughout the period of nursing.

REMEDIES. *Lycopodium*, *Sulphur*, *Natrum muriaticum*, *Carbo vegetabilis*, and *Calcarea carbonica*, have been employed with much success.

Dose.—Six globules of the appropriate remedy, every two or three days.

OF THE LOCHIA.

The discharges which take place after delivery are called lochia. If the quantity be excessive, it is similar to hemorrhage or flooding, and in that case see the remedies for flooding after delivery. After the first day or two, until about the tenth day, these discharges in appearance and quantity are something like the discharge of menstruation.

In a majority of cases, the red color leaves about the tenth day, and a yellowish discharge follows for a few days, which is often succeeded in its turn by a whitish or mucous discharge. After the woman begins to move about the house, the lochial discharge is apt to be renewed for a few days, and then takes its final leave.

If the lochia continue too long, or should be too profuse and full red, give *Aconite*, in water night and morning for two days. But, if that should not be sufficient, give *Calcarea carbonica* twice, dry. If it still continue, consult the remedies for flooding after delivery.

Bryonia, for suppression of the lochia with headache; fullness and heaviness of the head, with pressure in the forehead and temples; throbbing pains in the head, increased by motion; backache, with scanty emission of hot urine.

Dose.—Six globules dissolved in a teaspoonful of water, night and morning.

Platina, if the suppression be the result of some mental emotion, with dryness and over-sensitiveness of the sexual organs.

Dose.—Four globules three times a day.

Pulsatilla, if the suppression be sudden, from any accidental cause, with feverish excitement, with or without thirst; one-sided headache; oppression of the chest; partial heat of the upper part of the body, with coldness of feet; frequent inclination to pass water; the symptoms being worse in the evening, and better in the morning. This remedy is also suitable for a diminution, if there be not an entire suppression of the discharge.

Dose.—Dissolve twelve globules in a tumbler half full of water, and give a teaspoonful three or four times a day.

Rhus toxicodendron, for a variety of unhealthy lochiæ, if the discharge be offensive, black and watery, with shootings up the rectum; sharp pains shooting through the head, which feels as if it were too large; the head is worse when lying, and better after rising.

Dose.—The same as directed for Bryonia.

INFLAMMATION OF THE WOMB, OR METRITIS.

Diagnosis, external tension, with continuous pricking, burning, tumefaction, and acute shooting pain in the hypogastric region, with a sense of weight; the pain being increased by pressure upon the part. On examination there will be found heat and pain in the vagina; acute sensibility of the mouth of the womb, with suppression of the utero-vaginal secretions, and pain on passing urine, with constipation of the bowels.

CAUSES. Difficult labors, retention of the placenta.

version of the uterus, maltreatment, the use of stimulants; or it may be brought on by taking cold.

REMEDIES. *Aconite*, *Belladonna*, *Arnica*, *Nux vomica*, *Mercurius*, *Chamomilla*, *Coffea*, and *China*.

Aconite will be found useful in the commencement of this disease, where there is violent fever; or if the attack was caused by fright after confinement, or the abuse of chamomile tea.

Dose.—Dissolve twelve globules in a tumbler half full of water, and of this solution give a teaspoonful every two hours.

Belladonna, if the inflammation take place soon after confinement, with adherence of the placenta, or suppression of the discharges; burning pain in the hypogastrium, heaviness and drawing towards the genital organs, with aggravation from contact and motion.

Dose.—The same as for Aconite.

Arnica, if the inflammation should be the result of an injury, it may be given in alternation with Aconite.

Dose.—The same as for Aconite.

Nux vomica, aching pain in the region of the womb, increased by pressure or touch, with constipation, or hardened fæces in the rectum; swelling of the mouth of the womb, with sore pain, as if bruised internally.

Dose.—Six globules every two hours.

Mercurius, where there is frequent perspiration, or shuddering, with chills creeping up the back, and the pains are of a shooting or boring character.

Dose.—Six globules every two hours.

Chamomilla, if the inflammation is brought on by a fit of passion, or disappointment after confinement, with copious secretion of lochia, and discharge of dark, clotted blood.

Dose.—The same as directed for Aconite.

Coffea, when the attack arises from excessive or sudden joy during confinement, accompanied with fever and great restlessness.

Dose.—The same as for Mercurius.

China will be found useful in debilitated persons, or persons who have lost much blood, with spasmodic pains in the womb.

Dose.—The same as given for Belladonna.

INFLAMMATION OF THE OVARIES, OR OVARITIS.

Inflammation of the ovaries is characterized by shooting or pulsating pain in the iliac regions; also felt upon pressure; and may occur at any time, but more particularly soon after delivery; or it may arise in unmarried females, from undue excitement or excesses; upon examination, per vaginam or rectum, should there be much inflammation, a circumscribed swelling will be clearly perceived. In the acute form, the disease is attended with fever, headache, and gastric disturbance, hot feeling or itching in the vagina, and at times pain in the thighs, and difficulty in passing urine.

REMEDIES. *Aconite*, *Bryonia*, *Lachesis*, *Cantharis*, *Belladonna*, *Rhus toxicodendron*, *China*, and *Arsenicum album*.

Aconite may be given where there is a high degree of fever and inflammation.

Dose.—Five or six globules every three hours until the inflammatory symptoms have subsided, after which, select another remedy according to the remaining symptoms.

Bryonia, if the pain should be worse on movement, with pain in the limbs.

Dose.—The same as directed for Aconite.

Lachesis, in induration and suppuration of the ovaries.—(HERING.)

Cantharis, where there is difficulty in urinating, with burning pain, and pressing towards the genital organs.

Dose.—Six globules every six or eight hours until relief is afforded.

Belladonna, where there is a feeling upon pressure, as if bruised or beaten, with oppression of the chest, and palpitation of the heart.

Dose.—The same as directed for Aconite.

Rhus toxicodendron may be given with great benefit, where rest produces aggravation of all the symptoms.

Dose.—The same as directed for Aconite.

China, should there be indurations, or a dropsical tendency, with distension of the abdomen, or a feeling of fullness and pressing towards the genital organs.

Dose.—Four globules every six hours.

Arsenicum may be used if the pains become so violent as to cause the patient to toss about in agony, with writhing pain, alleviated by moving about.

Dose.—The same as of Belladonna.

COMING OF THE MILK.

Except in very few instances, the mother has no milk at the time of the birth of the child Milk generally makes its appearance on the third day, sometimes earlier and sometimes later. Previous to the formation of milk, the breasts enlarge more or less, and sometimes to such an extent as to give rise to a great deal of suffering, especially with first children. Care should be taken not to bruise the breasts at this time by rudely rubbing them, or officiousness in drawing them, in order to get out the "caked" milk. The state of turgescence, which precedes the secretion of milk, is widely different, and must be distinguished from the state of distension of the breasts, which follows the secretion.

Aconite, if the breasts be hard and knotted; dry and hot skin; redness of the face; the patient is restless and discouraged.

Dose.—Dissolve twelve globules in a tumbler half full of water, and give a teaspoonful every three or four hours.

Bryonia should be given after Aconite, if that remedy mitigates the symptoms but does not remove them, or, if some of them disappear and others remain.

Dose.—The same as directed for Aconite.

Belladonna may be given after Bryonia, or alternately with it, if a portion of the same group of symptoms still continue.

Dose.—The same as directed for Aconite.

Calcarea carbonica is especially suitable if there be a deficiency in the secretion of milk in the out-set, or fullness or enlargement of the breasts, with tardiness in the formation of milk. This remedy is also most important when the milk runs out too easy.

Dose. -Six globules dissolved in a teaspoonful of water, three times a day.

Chamomilla is suitable if there be excessive sensibility of the nervous system, with restlessness; tenderness of the breasts; and inflammation of the nipples, so that the milk cannot run out.

Dose.—The same as directed for Aconite.

Pulsatilla, when the secretion of milk is interrupted, or entirely suppressed; threatening symptoms of child-bed fever. This medicine exercises a healthful influence over the female constitution, in almost every deviation from the natural course, during the entire period of nursing. It is also very effectual in re-establishing the equilibrium of the organism at the time of weaning.

Dose.—Six globules four times a day, dissolved in a teaspoonful of water.

Rhus toxicodendron, in painful distension of the breasts, with rheumatic pains throughout the system; swelling, heat, and hardness of the breasts, causing headache, stiffness of the joints, and other constitutional disturbance. Rhus toxicodendron is very serviceable in warding off the ill consequences of a suppression of milk, and also at the time of weaning.

Dose.—The same as Calcarea carbonica.

As local applications, I frequently direct the

breasts to be bathed with hot lard, and then enveloped in raw cotton.

SORE NIPPLES.

Arnica, in the form of lotion, made by dissolving five drops of the tincture in a wineglassful of water, and bathing the nipples several times a day, is very effectual in removing the tenderness and excoriation consequent upon the first few applications of the child's mouth. Be careful to moisten the nipple with saliva or mucilage, before giving it to the child.

Chamomilla, for inflammation, swelling, and ulceration of the nipples.

Dose.—Four globules dissolved in a teaspoonful of water, three times a day.

Graphites, for burning, aching, cracking, and tenderness of the nipples.

Dose.—Four globules night and morning in a little water.

Sulphur, when the nipples are sore and deeply chapped; the chaps bleed, and burn like fire; deep fissure around the base of the nipples.

Dose.—The same as directed for Chamomilla.

In difficult cases one of the following medicines may be given alternately, with Sulphur, night and morning, viz: *Calcarea carbonica*, *Lycopodium*, *Mercurius vivus*, or *Silicea*.

GATHERED BREASTS.

During the entire period of lactation, the breasts are more or less liable to inflammation and suppuration. Abscesses sometimes form, from mechanical injuries and needless exposure, in the breasts of unmarried women.

Belladonna is indicated if the breasts be swollen and hard, with shooting and tearing pains, and redness which radiates from a central point.

Dose.—Four globules dissolved in a teaspoonful of water, four times a day.

Bryonia, when the breasts are too full of milk, hard, and feel heavy, like the weight of a stone, with shooting pains; dry skin and other feverish symptoms. Bryonia and Belladonna can frequently be given alternately, with very great advantage.

Dose.—The same as directed for Belladonna.

Hepar sulphur, after the administration of Belladonna and Bryonia, if the swelling continue, and especially if throbbings make their appearance.

Dose.—Dissolve eight globules in a wineglassful of water, and give a teaspoonful every three or four hours.

Phosphorus, when the foregoing remedies have not been sufficient to arrest the progress of the inflammation, but suppuration having established itself, the abscess is discharged through fistulous openings which are not disposed to heal.

Dose.—The same as of Belladonna.

Sulphur, if the discharge of matter be profuse, with chilliness through the forenoon, and feverish heat with flushed cheeks in the afternoon.

Dose.—Six globules three times a day.

STATE OF THE BOWELS.

It is perfectly natural for the bowels to remain without being moved, for a few days after delivery. In a majority of cases, the bowels move about the fifth day. In no case should purgative medicine be given during confinement. If headache, pain in the bowels, or other symptoms of costiveness appear, give one dose of Bryonia in the evening and another in the morning. Should there be no change by the following evening, give a dose of Nux vomica in water, and a dose of Sulphur next morning. Should these remedies not procure an evacuation, and the unpleasant symptoms remain, give an injection of luke-warm water.

If diarrhœa should occur during confinement, *Dulcamara*, *Phosphoric acid*, *Rheum* or *Veratrum*, will be found to control it without difficulty.

Dose.—Dissolve twenty globules of the appropriate remedy in eight teaspoonsful of water, andtake a teaspoonful after each evacuation until the diarrhœa ceases.

RETENTION OF URINE AFTER DELIVERY.

Frequently after delivery, especially with first children, and in protracted or tedious labors, there is retention or painful emissions of urine. One of the following remedies will generally suffice to procure a free emission, or sitting over a chamber which contains warm water is sometimes useful: *Arnica*, *Belladonna*, *Nux vomica*, and *Pulsatilla.*

Arnica, where retention has been caused by difficult labor, and there is much soreness of the parts; tenesmus of the neck of the bladder; desire to urinate, with burning pain; stitches in the urethra; urine brown, with brick-red sediment.

Dose.—Four globules three times a day will generally remove all unpleasant symptoms.

Belladonna, frequent desire to urinate, which is passed with difficulty; urine yellow and turbid; painful constriction of the neck of the bladder.

Dose.—Four globules every four or six hours, until relief is obtained.

Nux vomica, painful ineffectual desire to urinate, with burning and lacerating pain in the neck of the bladder; nightly urging to urinate, with violent burning.

Dose.—The same as directed for Belladonna.

Pulsatilla will be of great use where there is

catarrh of the bladder, with frequent, almost ineffectual urging to urinate, with pressure as from a stone; spasmodic pain in the neck of the bladder, extending to the thighs.

Dose.—Six globules dissolved in half a tumbler of water, and a teaspoonful to be taken every three hours.

In case the above treatment should not succeed in 18 or 24 hours, and the retention become painful, the urine must be drawn off by means of the catheter.

DURATION OF CONFINEMENT.

For the first four or five days after delivery, a woman should remain quiet in bed, keep her mind free from excitement, and live on gruel, panada, toast and black tea, or other similar articles, and drink cold water. Afterwards, should no untoward symptoms be present, she may rise daily to have her bed made, and gradually return to her ordinary diet. The first two weeks should be chiefly spent in bed, or at least in the recumbent posture, during which time visiters ought not to be admitted. A woman ought not to leave her room before three weeks, and never go up or down stairs before four weeks after her confinement.

PART II.

TREATMENT OF CHILDREN.

TREATMENT OF CHILDREN.

RECEPTION AT BIRTH.

In case a child is born before the arrival of the accoucheur, some person should place it in a proper position to breathe; and if the cord be coiled round the neck, body, or limbs of the child, it should be disengaged, in order that the circulation between the mother and child may not be interrupted before respiration is fully established in the latter. Remove the child a little out of the discharges, so that the face at least may be free, and if the mouth or nostrils are obstructed by mucus, cleanse them with a napkin, or piece of fine linen, wrapped round the little finger. When these things are attended to, if the child be healthy and robust, it will cry lustily; and its skin will change from a light or leaden hue, to a pink or rose color. There is now no further cause for alarm, as both mother and child may remain in this situation for an hour or two without danger. If, however, the child should be feeble, or have been delayed long in the birth, or either of the causes above mentioned have operated to prevent it from breathing, and after the above directions shall have been followed respiration do not yet take place, wrap the child's body and limbs in warm flannel or napkins, and apply cold water, or cold spirits, to its breast, with the palm of the hand; should this not succeed, place your mouth over the child's mouth, and gently blow so as to inflate the lungs, closing the child's nostrils at the same time between your thumb and finger, to keep the air from passing out through its nose. If pulsation be felt in the cord, and the beating of the child's heart be perceptible, have a little patience and all will be well.

After respiration is fully established with the child, and pulsation have ceased in the cord, and not before, the child may be removed. In order to do this, take a string made of sewing thread doubled and twisted, which is best; or, in place of that, a piece of narrow tape, or round bobbin of sufficient strength, will answer. Wrap the string *once* round the cord, about an inch and a half from the child's stomach, and tie it securely in a hard knot; cut off the loose ends of the string, and tie one of them round the cord three-quarters of an inch farther up, and then cut the cord with a pair of scissors between the two ligatures.

The child may be received in a blanket or sheet, which should be warmed for the purpose.

ASPHYXIA, OR APPARENT DEATH OF NEW-BORN INFANTS.

This condition of new-born children is generally caused by the winding of the cord around the neck; by long detention of the head in the pelvis; by tedious labors; the accumulation of mucus in the mouth and throat; sudden change of temperature before respiration is fully established, &c.

REMEDIES. *Tartar emetic*, *Aconite*, *China*, and *Opium*.

Tartar emetic may be given where there are no signs of life, slight pulsations of the cord, or if the face is purple and swollen.

Dose.—Dissolve six globules in four tablespoonsful of water, and of this solution give six drops every few minutes, until there are signs of life.

Aconite, when life is restored, and when the face has previously been of a bluish color.

Dose.—Two globules every ten or fifteen minutes, until complete restoration has taken place.

China, for similar symptoms, as for Aconite, except where the face has been pale.

Dose.—The same as of Aconite.

Opium may be used if Tartar emetic fails to produce any beneficial effect in fifteen or twenty minutes, especially if the face has a bluish appearance.

Dose.—The same as of Aconite.

WASHING THE CHILD.

The body of almost every new-born babe is more or less covered with a white unctuous matter, which adheres to it with great tenacity. The best method of removing it is by rubbing the covered parts of the child freely with hogs' lard, until the two substances become completely incorporated, when they are easily removed by a piece of flannel, which should always be used as a wash-rag. When the skin is freed from the unctuous matter, a little fine soap may be used, to get rid of the grease. After the child has been carefully washed, which should be well done the first time, its skin should be rendered perfectly dry with a fine napkin. The reprehensible practice of bathing children in spirits, should always be prohibited.

DRESSING OF THE NAVEL.

This is to be done, by folding a piece of linen or muslin, until it is about six inches long, and three wide, consisting of four or six thicknesses, in which a hole is to be cut, and the cord passed through. The cord is then to have another strip of linen or muslin wrapped round it, as you would wrap up a sore finger. The first piece of linen or muslin lying lengthwise of the child's body, the end of the cord now wrapped is to be laid up towards the child's breast, and the lower end of the first piece is to be folded over it, and the whole secured by the belly-band, which should always be made of a strip of flannel, without either heming or lining. The navel usually comes off from the fifth to the eighth day.

OF THE MECONIUM.

In most cases the child's bowels are moved a few hours after birth. The substance discharged is of a dark bottle-green color, and is called meconium. To aid the discharge of the meconium, and to clear the throat of mucus, it is allowable to give the child two or three teaspoonsful of warm water, sweetened with brown sugar. The first milk has a tendency to promote the object. The color of the stools generally changes to yellow about the fifth day.

If the bowels should not be moved as freely, or as frequently in the few first days as they ought to be, and the child be restless, give four globules of Nux vomica at night, and if necessary, the same of Chamomilla the next day.

LOCK-JAW OF INFANTS.

This serious disease is almost exclusively confined to tropical climates, and happens only in the first days of infantile life. The child cries, and in vain attempts to nurse, the milk chokes it, and is ejected. On examination, the masseter muscles are found to be so rigid, that the lower jaw cannot be depressed; the jaws gradually close, the abdomen swells, the stiffness extends to the whole frame, and in two or three days the little sufferer is relieved by death. It is generally caused by foul atmosphere, taking cold, improper food, and local irritation from mechanical causes.

REMEDIES. *Arnica*, *Belladonna*, *Chamomilla*, *Mercurius vivus*, and *Lachesis*.

Arnica, if it has been caused by mechanical injuries, irritation about the umbilicus, &c.

Dose.—Three globules every four hours, at the same time, linen cloths wet with a solution, made of ten drops of the tincture of Arnica to a wineglassfull of water, may be applied locally.

Belladonna, where it cannot be assigned to any particular cause, and the child cannot swallow.

Dose.—Three globules every hour.

Chamomilla, if it has been brought on by a sudden chill or fright.

Dose.—Four globules every two hours.

Mercurius may be given, if Belladonna has failed to give relief.

Dose.—The same as Belladonna.

Lachesis, if it is caused by a bad state of the mother's milk.

Dose.—Four globules every three hours.

PUTTING THE CHILD TO THE BREAST.

After the lapse of ten or twelve hours, or sooner if the mother have milk, the child may be put to the breast, after carefully moistening the nipple as before directed. In a majority of cases, it is best to comply with the above direction for the reasons, that it learns the child to suck, softens the nipple, and invites an early flow of milk. The mother's milk is the most natural food for the child, but when this cannot be procured, and a substitute becomes necessary, we ought to imitate it as near as we can. For this purpose, take fresh milk from one cow, add one-third warm water, and sweeten it with a little loaf sugar. Of this, a child may take a few teaspoonsful at a time, as often as may be necessary. Never give a new-born infant cracker victuals, gruel, pap, panada, or other cooked food. Every infant should have a teaspoonful or two of cold water given to it every day, or several times a day, if the water agrees with it.

REGURGITATION OF MILK.

Children, during the period of nursing, frequently overload their stomach, and regurgitate some of the milk; thus far, mothers need feel no uneasiness, nor is medical aid required, but should the nutriment be ejected from the stomach by vomiting, or if it should occur in children who have been weaned, it must be treated according to its symptoms.

REMEDIES. *Ipecacuanha*, *Pulsatilla*, *Bryonia*, *Nux vomica*, and *Chamomilla.*

Ipecacuanha will mostly give relief, especially in children who have been overfed, and where the food taken is of such a nature as to disagree with the stomach or if diarrhœa or flatulency be present.

Dose.—Four globules every hour or two, until the child is relieved.

Pulsatilla, when there is diarrhœa, with a fit of crying, and the food is not easily digested.

Dose.—Four globules every four hours.

Bryonia and *Nux vomica*, where there is a tendency to constipation, with irritable disposition and uneasiness.

Dose.—The same as for Pulsatilla.

Chamomilla, should the disease be accompanied

with diarrhœa or convulsions, and where the attack is attended at the onset by fever or colic, with great restlessness.

Dose.—Four globules every fifteen, twenty, or thirty minutes, according to the circumstances of the case.

ELONGATION OF THE HEAD.

In first children, and after other tedious and protracted labors, it is common to find a tumor on the back of the child's head, giving it the appearance of being elongated. The repeated application of cold water, with a few drops of the tincture of Arnica dissolved in it, will remove the trouble in a few days.

HICCOUGH, OR SINGULTUS.

This is a common and mostly unimportant affection, and may generally be left altogether to nature. But if it should become troublesome, so as to prevent sleep, two or three globules of Ignatia or Pulsatilla put on the tongue will relieve it.

INFLAMMATION OF THE EYES.

Very young infants are subject to inflammation of the eyes; sometimes the lids only are affected, at other times the lids and eye-balls are both involved. The eyes should not be exposed to too strong a light, and the child should be kept out of every draft of air; as light and cold are the most common, although not the only causes of the disease.

REMEDIES. *Aconite*, *Belladonna*, *Chamomilla*, *Euphrasia*, and *Rhus toxicodendron.*

Aconite, when cold or exposure to the light is the cause; when the whole eye is very red, and runs a great deal.

Dose.—Six globules dissolved in a tumbler half full of water, and a teaspoonful of the solution to be taken every two or three hours, according to the violence of the inflammation.

Belladonna, when the whites of the eyes are very red, and present a blood-shot appearance; or there is bleeding from the eye-lids, and the child cannot bear the light.

Dose.—The same as directed for Aconite.

Chamomilla, if the eyes bleed, are swollen, and are closed in the morning.

Dose.—Four globules three times a day, dissolved in a teaspoonful of water.

Euphrasia, when the eyes are very much gummed up, and run acrid yellow water; and the child cannot bear the light.

Dose.—The same as directed for Aconite.

Rhus toxicodendron is very important in scrofulous children, and where the lids are principally affected.

Dose.—Four globules night and morning.

In addition to the above treatment the following remedies will also, at times, be found very useful: *Hepar sulphur*, *Mercurius vivus*, *Sulphur*, *Nux vomica*, and *Arsenicum*.

Hepar sulphur may be used in obstinate cases, especially where large quantities of Mercury have been used, and the symptoms should indicate a complication of mercurial and natural disease.

Dose.—Six globules dissolved in a tumbler half full of water, and a teaspoonful of the solution to be taken, morning, noon, and night.

Mercurius vivus will be found useful in a purely syphilitic form of this affection, and will in the majority of cases effect a speedy cure, after which a few doses of Sulphur may be requisite to control the excessive secretion of mucus.

Dose.—Six globules in a teaspoonful of water three times a day.

Surphur, this is an important remedy in all kinds of inflammation of the eyes, when of an obstinate or inveterate character, especially where there is an excessive secretion of mucus; also, where there is pressure; burning or smarting pain, as if from sand; itching in the eyes or eyelids.

Dose.—Six globules in a teaspoonful of water night and morning.

Nux vomica, if there are burning, pressive or aching pains, with stiffness, smarting or itching; slight fever morning and evening; the eyes blood-shot and swollen, with adhesion of the eyelids; sensibility to the light; affection worse towards morning.

Dose.—Four globules in a teaspoonful of water every six hours.

Arsenicum, if there is violent burning pain, with swelling of the lids; dark redness and congestion of the vessels, especially if the inflammation is of a scrofulous character.

Dose.—The same as directed for Sulphur.

SNIFFLES.

Infants are often attacked with a kind of catarrh, or obstruction of the nose, which prevents them from breathing whilst they are sucking.

REMEDIES. *Nux vomica*, *Sambucus*, and *Chamomilla*.

Nux vomica, where there is oppressive dullness of the head, continual heat and dryness of the nose, or fluent coryza in the day-time, and dry coryza at night.

Dose.—Four globules dissolved in a wineglass of water, and a teaspoonful to be given three times a day, and if no relief is obtained in twenty-four hours, give the next mentioned remedy.

Sambucus, if there is stoppage of the nose, with accumulation of thick, tenacious mucus.

Dose.—The same as directed for Nux vomica.

Chamomilla will be found very useful, if there

is a watery discharge from the nose, or if the nostrils are sore and ulcerated.

Dose.—Three globules every four hours until better.

SORE MOUTH.

Baby's sore mouth, is also called Thrush and Aphthæ. It runs in families, and is apt to make its appearance towards the latter end of the second week. Much may be done to prevent this troublesome complaint, by proper attention to cleanliness. A child should be thoroughly washed every day, in slightly tepid water, and the mouth cleansed with cold water on a piece of fine linen rag, and afterwards the child should be allowed to suck the rag wet with the cold water.

REMEDIES. *Mercurius vivus*, *Sulphur*, *Bryonia*, and *Nux vomica.*

Mercurius vivus, where there is inflammation of the whole bucal cavity; ptyalism, with apthous ulcers in the mouth, which readily become gangrenous; gums swollen and ulcerated.

Dose.—Give six globules night and morning, for two or three days, and if no improvement takes place, or the ulcers do not disappear, give the following remedy.

Sulphur, apthous vesicles in the mouth, with burning pain; heat in the mouth, with much thirst at night; burning pain on the surface of the tongue.

Dose.—The same as directed for Mercurius vivus.

Bryonia, where there is dryness of the mouth with great thirst; burning vescicles on the edge of the tongue; the gums are painful, sore, and spongy

Dose.—Four globules dissolved in a teaspoonful of water, night and morning until better.

Nux vomica, fetid ulcers in the mouth, and fæces; painful vescicles on the tongue, which is coated with white or yellow mucus.

Dose.—The same as directed for Bryonia.

The common domestic remedy is equal parts of Borax and loaf-sugar finely pulverized, and a pinch of it put into the child's mouth three or four times a day. In many cases it answers very well, but it should not be pushed too far.

JAUNDICE.

The skin of children for some time after birth being very delicate and vascular, is consequently much redder than it is when they are more advanced. During the transition from the red to a paler color, the skin often assumes a yellowness, somewhat resembling jaundice; but this does not constitute the disease. This yellow tint may continue for a few days, without being attended by any other symptoms, and then disappear spontaneously. Although the skin be yellow, if the child is not sick, and the secretions be natural, there is no need of medicine.

But, if in addition to the yellowness of the skin, the whites of the eyes, the secretion of tears and urine be yellow, and the evacuation from the bowels be paler than natural, or of a clay color; if the abdomen swell; if the child be fretful and moan frequently, there need be no further delay: the child is sick, and requires treatment.

REMEDIES. *Chamomilla* and *Mercurius vivus.*

Chamomilla, where there is sleeplessness; cries and starting in the sleep; dryness of the mouth, and heat of the face, and there are discharges of whtie mucus from the bowels.

Dose.—Three globules three times a day until better.

Mercurius vivus may be used in alternation with, or follow Chamomilla, provided Chamomilla has failed to produce relief.

Dose.—The same as of Chamomilla.

If no relief has been obtained from the use of the above remedies, send for a homœopathic physician.

OF THE GUM.

This for the most part is an artificial disease. It consists of a crop of red pimples, more or less extensive and numerous; it generally occupies the face, neck, and arms; other parts also are visited by it. Bathe the child properly; do not keep it too warm, and give it no *saffron*, *sweet majorum* or *cat-nep* tea, and it will not be much troubled with the gum.

REMEDIES. *Rhus toxicodendron* and *Sulphur.*

Rhus toxicodendron will be found useful, if the eruption, consisting of small, red pimples, appears on the neck, arms, or loins, or if the vesicles are confluent, and contain a watery secretion.

Dose.—Four globules in a teaspoonful of water, night and morning.

Sulphur, where there is a fiery, scarlet eruption, which occasions violent itching and burning.

Dose.—Four globules night and morning.

RETENTION OF URINE.

Young infants are frequently the subjects of this complaint. Dissolve six pellets of *Aconite* in a wineglassful of water, and give the child a portion of it every two or three hours until relief is obtained. Should this fail, give *Nux vomica* or *Pulsatilla* in the same way.

PROFUSE URINATION.

Occasionally young children have frequent and profuse emissions of colorless and inodorous urine. They are apt to be pale and fretful during its continuance.

REMEDIES. *Phophoric acid* or *Silicea.*

Phosphoric acid, irresistible desire to urinate enuresis, with cutting and burning; frequent micturition; urine fetid.

Dose.—Three globules, morning, noon, and night.

Silicea, desire to urinate, with copious emission, especially at night, with smarting in the urethra.

Dose.—Three globules at night for two successive nights.

CONSTIPATION.

If the evacuations have the natural color and consistency, although they should not occur so frequently as would be desirable, it is not always the part of wisdom to interfere, by giving medicine. If left to themselves, they will often return to the natural state; but if collateral symptoms arise we must give medicine.

It often happens that the constipation or diarrhœa of a child depends upon the mother or the nurse, and in that case the medicine should be given to them, so as to operate on the child through the medium of the milk.

REMEDIES. *Bryonia*, *Calcarea carbonica*, *Nux vomica*, and *Opium.*

Bryonia, constipation, with hard, tough stool; or dry, as if burnt; or the fæces are large and passed with difficulty, with burning pain in the rectum after stool; or stool followed with diarrhœa.

Dose.—Six globules three times a day.

Calcarea carbonica, if there is hard, undigested stool; or constant urging without stool; or stool scanty and mixed with blood.

Dose.—The same as directed for Bryonia.

Nux vomica, constipation, as if from inactivity of the bowels; anxious and frequent ineffectual urging to stool; fæces large and hard.

Dose.—Three globules dissolved in a teaspoonful of water, night and morning.

Opium, hard stool; costiveness; nothing but small, hard balls being passed.

Dose.—The same as of Nux vomica.

DIARRHŒA.

The diarrhœa of infants will not always yield to the medicines which are successful at other periods.

REMEDIES. *Belladonna*, *Chamomilla*, and *Rheum*.

Belladonna, if the child sleeps a great deal, but is uneasy; paleness of the face; every time the child is changed, the napkin is found to be soiled by a small greenish discharge.

Dose.—Six globules dissolved in a wineglassful of water, and a easpoonful to be given every four hours.

Chamomilla, when the evacuations are watery

and greenish, or like beaten-up eggs, and worse at night; the stools are attended with straining, and redness of the child's face; frequent small green stools with restlessness.

Dose.—Six globules dissolved in a teaspoonful of water, morning, noon, and night.

Rheum, in diarrhœa arising from acidity, attended with cries, colic and straining; bearing down without stool; the evacuations are frothy, sometimes slimy, and smell sour; the child smells sour, notwithstanding the greatest attention to cleanliness.

Dose.—The same as directed for Chamomilla.

COLIC.

Infants, and especially those of feeble constitutions, are troubled with colic in the month. It may arise from constitutional peculiarity, or from improper feeding of the child, and from improprieties on the part of the mother—either errors of diet, exposure to cold, or suffering of any kind, that will interfere with the healthy secretion of milk. If the child's food disagrees with it, it is apt to exhibit signs of pain soon after feeding. The attacks may be so severe and frequent, as almost to wear out both mother and child. Diarrhœa frequently attends it.

There is another species of colic, to which some

of the most robust, and otherwise healthy children, are subject. It is periodical in its attacks, which usually occur at five or six o'clock in the afternoon. This species is often attended with costiveness, but frequently the state of the bowels is unchanged. The complaint does not interfere with the growth or general health of the child, and usually stops when the child is about three months old.

Whatever may be the cause of colic in children, it should be sought out, and if possible removed.

REMEDIES. *Chamomilla*, *China*, *Ipecacuanha*, and *Pulsatilla*.

Chamomilla, if the pain be attended with looseness of the bowels; yellowish green and watery discharges; distension of the abdomen; writhing pain; constant crying and drawing up of the legs, with coldness of the feet.

Dose.—Dissolve six globules in three tablespoonsful of water, and give a teaspoonful every fifteen or thirty minutes, according to the severity of the symptoms, until the child is relieved.

China, when the pains come on late in the afternoon, with hardness of the abdomen; the child screams, and laughs immediately afterwards; the bowels may be in a healthy state, or the stools may be whitish and curdled.

Dose.—The same as directed for Chamomilla.

Ipecacuanha, when the cries of the child are sharp, as if the pains were of the cutting kind; fermented stools of a putrid odor. This medicine is well adapted to the various ailments of the stomach and bowels of young children.

Dose.—Three globules dissolved in a teaspoonful of water, every two or three hours.

Pulsatilla, is very useful in flatulent colic, especially if it occur in the evening, or every other day, accompanied with shiverings and paleness of the face; rumbling of wind through the bowels, with tenderness of the abdomen.

Dose.—The same as directed for Ipecacuanha.

CRYING OF INFANTS.

An infant is not always in pain when it cries. This is the language by which it makes known its wants. It may be hungry or need changing. Young infants should never be obliged to lie in one position longer than an hour or two at a time. They should be placed on the side to sleep, and turned over occasionally.

Although the above be true, we are not to think that children never have pain when they cry. An experienced ear can generally perceive a difference in the tone, and in that way determine whether the child have pain or not. If a child continue to cry and will not be pacified, the cause should be diligently sought for—a pin may be pricking it, or its clothes may be too tight, or it may have pain somewhere.

REMEDIES. *Belladonna*, *Aconite*, *Coffea*, and *Chamomilla.*

Belladonna, if the child continues to cry for a long time without any apparent cause, or starts out of its sleep and cries.

Dose.—Dissolve six globules in half a tumblerful of water, and give a teaspoonful every one, two, or three hours, according to circumstances.

Aconite, if there be much uneasiness, accompanied with dry heat.

Dose.—The same as directed for Belladonna.

Coffea, if the child appears to be nervous and very restless, with heat, and tossing about.

Dose.—Three globules every hour until it is better.

Chamomilla, when the child cries, and is restless, with frequent startings, or there is reason to believe it has earache or headache, and cries when it is moved.

Dose.—The same as directed for Belladonna.

RESTLESSNESS AND WAKEFULNESS.

Restlessness and inability to sleep are generally produced by injurious food being given to the child, or by the mother drinking green tea and coffee, or using other improper articles of diet.

REMEDIES. *Belladonna*, *Chamomilla*, *Coffea*, and *Opium*.

Belladonna, if the child seems inclined to sleep, and cannot sleep, but starts up and cries.

Dose.—Dissolve eight globules in a wineglassful of water, and give a teaspoonful every half hour.

Chamomilla, if the sleeplessness be attended with flatulency, with starts and jerkings of the limbs; or feverish heat, with redness of one cheek.

Dose.—The same as directed for Belladonna.

Coffea, if there be increased heat of the body, with great nervous excitability.

Dose.—Three globules every half hour until better.

Opium, if no relief is obtained after several doses of the preceding remedy, and the face is red.

Dose.—The same as of Coffea.

SWELLING OF THE BREASTS.

At birth, or very soon afterwards, the breasts of infants are sometimes found to be swollen. A common opinion prevails among nurses and others, that this swelling and inflammation is owing to the presence of milk, which must be squeezed out before they can get well. This opinion is not true

—there is no milk there, neither do the breasts require squeezing. By rude handling, the inflammation is sometimes urged on to suppuration—matter is formed, and in some instances the breasts have been destroyed, and females deprived of their usefulness for ever.

In most cases, there is nothing more necessary than to apply a piece of linen wet with sweet oil to them. In a few severe cases it may be necessary to apply a bread and milk poultice, and renew it as occasion may require.

REMEDIES. *Chamomilla*, *Belladonna*, *Hepar sulphur*, and *Calcarea curbonica.*

Chamomilla, if there is extensive swelling of the breasts, attended with redness and inflammation.

Dose.—Four globules dissolved in a teaspoonful of water, three times a day.

Belladonna, if the breasts are swollen, hard, and painful.

Dose.—The same as directed for Chamomilla.

Hepar sulphur will be indicated, should formation of matter have taken place.

Dose.—Dissolve six globules in eight teaspoonsful of water, and give a teaspoonful every four hours.

Silicea, should Hepar sulphur be insufficient to stop the formation of matter.

Dose.—The same as directed for Hepar sulphur.

EXCORIATIONS.

Unless there be strong predisposition to excoriations, proper attention to cleanliness, and care being taken to dry all the creases in fat children after washing, they will very generally be prevented. A child that is kept so warm as to make it perspire a great deal, is very liable to excoriations.

When they take place, the child should be washed in luke-warm water (without soap), and made dry by the repeated application of a fine linen handkerchief without rubbing. Afterwards it should be powdered with finely pulverized wheaten starch. Although excoriations are sometimes bad to look at, they are not dangerous, and a little patience and close attention will overcome them.

While the above directions are being followed externally, one or more of the following medicines may be administered internally, namely: *Carbo vegetabilis*, *Chamomilla*, *Lycopodium*, *Mercurius vivus*, or *Sulphur*.

Carbo vegetabilis, if there is much rawness of the parts affected, or where there is a general disposition in the parts to become excoriated.

Dose.—Six globules night and morning.

Chamomilla, if the skin become easily exco

riated, with burning, smarting, and great sensitiveness of the touch.

Dose.—Four globules three times a day.

Lycopodium, if the skin of the whole body is dry and hot, and cracks èasily, with violent itching when heated.

Dose.—Four globules night and morning.

Mercurius vivus, violent itching of the skin—worse at night—aggravated by the heat of the bed.

Dose.—The same as directed for Chamomilla.

Sulphur, itching of the skin of the whole body; scurfy eruption; soreness of the skin of infants.

Dose.—Dissolve six globules in a wineglassful of water, and give teaspoonful night and morning.

SCURF ON THE HEAD.

Children that are kept too warm, or that are a little neglected, are liable to have an unsightly, dirty-looking incrustation formed on the top of the head. On removing any part of the crust, the skin beneath will be found red and inflamed. It annoys the child by its itching, and others by its offensiveness. The forcible removal of it by the fine-tooth comb will not effect a cure, for so long as the diseased state of the scalp remains, it will be speedily reproduced.

It can be prevented by washing the child's head regularly every morning, and after drying it properly, using a suitable hair brush.

If a tendency to this formation be noticed, give the child *Staphysagria* two nights in succession.

Dose.—Six globules dissolved in a teaspoonful of water.

After the crust has formed, it can be removed by anointing it well with lard at night, and washing it off next morning with a solution of *Borax* in water. The application may have to be repeated three or four times.

CRUSTA LACTEA, OR MILK CRUST.

This eruption, to which infants are liable, consists of small, whitish vesicles, or blisters, that appear in clusters upon a red ground. The vesicles burst and form yellow scabs, from beneath which a straw-colored, watery fluid issues. The eruption commences generally upon one cheek, from whence it extends to the adjacent portions of the face and scalp. The swelling of the scalp is sometimes considerable, and the itching is frequently intense, causing great restlessness of the child. Scratching aggravates the disease and causes the eruption to bleed.

REMEDIES. *Aconite*, *Rhus toxicodendron*, *Sulphur*, *Arsenicum*, *Graphites*, *Sepia*, *Lycopodium*, and *Viola tricolor*.

Aconite, in the very commencement of the disease, where there is dry, hot skin, fever, great restlessness and excitability, and the skin is inflamed, with itching.

Dose.—Three globules every four hours.

Rhus toxicodendron, itching, burning vesicles, with red, inflamed base; or pustules filled with a watery fluid, attended with violent itching and swelling of the lower parts.

Dose.—Four globules three times a day.

Sulphur, scabby, tettery eruption, with violent itching, or where there is no disposition in the eruption to dry up; it may be given in alternation with Rhus toxicodendron.

Dose.—Four globules twice a day.

Arsenicum, in complicated cases, or where the eruption bursts and ulcerates, attended with the sensation of burning.

Dose.—Six globules three times a day.

Graphites, in tettery eruptions, generally small pimples like flea-bites, with dryness of the skin and itching of the hairy scalp, with falling off of the hair.

Dose.—Six globules night and morning.

Sepia, excoriation, with brown, red, or tettery

eruptions, or running sores, with itching and burning.

Dose.—Six globules twice a day.

Lycopodium, in tedious cases, where there is itching and much matter discharged, with swelling of the glands of the neck.

Dose.—Four globules night and morning.

Viola tricolor, scabs on the face and head, with thick incrustations, with burning itching at night, and discharge of thick, yellow matter.

Dose.—Six globules night and morning.

SCALD HEAD, OR TINEA CAPITIS; OR WHITE RINGWORM OF THE SCALP.

This is a disease of the hairy portion of the scalp, which mostly appears from the first to the twelfth year of age, and is characterized by the following symptoms: The child complains of an itching, burning pain on parts of the head, where small, round, pointed efflorescences on an inflamed rose-colored ground make their appearance, which are hard at their base, but soft and yellowish at their points. They gradually become more elevated, burst, and give rise to a viscous, acrid, offensive discharge—thus extending the disease to the parts with which it comes in contact. The hair becomes matted and scaley; hard crusts are formed, from beneath which the secretion of matter continues. The disease is usually attended with swelling of the glands of the head and neck.

REMEDIES. *Rhus toxicodendron*, *Dulcamara*, *Bryonia*, *Staphysagria*, *Hepar sulphur*, *Arsenicum*, *Antimonium crudum*, *Calcarea carbonica*, *Sulphur*, *Graphites*, and *Lycopodium*.

Rhus toxicodendron is recommended where there is much itching, burning, and where the patches are inflamed and irritable.

Dose.—Six globules twice a day.

Dulcamara, if it is attended with hard swelling of the glands of the throat and neck, with pale face, and loose, flabby muscles.

Dose.—Six globules twice a day

Bryonia, when the glands are painful, red, hard, and swollen.

Dose.—The same as Dulcamara.

Staphysagria, if the eruption is moist, with itching and offensive discharge.

Dose.—Four globules three times daily.

Hepar sulphur, if the eruption extends from the head to other parts, as the face, neck; or the eyes become inflamed and swollen, and ulceration behind the ears take place.

Dose.—Four globules three times a day.

Arsenicum, if other remedies afford no relief, and

the discharge becomes acrid and offensive, with a disposition to ulceration.

Dose.—Four globules twice a day.

Antimonium crudum, if the eruption extends over the whole face, and thick scabs form on the head, with violent itching.

Dose.—Six globules three times a day.

Calcarea carbonica, in those of scrofulous taint, especially fat children with light complexion, and with swelling of the glands of the neck, and with falling out of the hair.

Dose.—Six globules twice a day.

Sulphur, when the eruption commences to dry and the scabs begin to scale off.

Dose.—Six globules night and morning.

Graphites, scabs with itching of the hairy scalp; humid eruption on the head, which is painful to the touch, with the feeling as if ulcerated.

Dose.—Six globules every night.

Lycopodium, eruption on the head, with fetid, profuse suppuration, and violent itching of the hairy scalp.

Dose.—Six globules every night.

INFANTILE ERYSIPELAS.

Infants within the first two months of their lives are sometimes attacked with a kind of erysipelas of the surface, attended with hardness and swelling underneath. It is mostly located on the nates or genital organs, but may attack other parts, and go on to suppuration. When it attacks the maxillary muscles, the child cannot cry. It appears first in the form of red spots, attended with general fever, hot skin, and thirst. In the latter stage of the disease, there is a characteristic dryness and harshness of the skin, almost like parchment.

REMEDIES. *Aconite*, *Belladonna*, *Rhus toxicodendron*, *Arsenicum* and *Sulphur*.

Aconite, in the beginning, when there is fever, thirst, and dry skin.

Dose.—Four globules every four hours.

Belladonna, if there is fever, and the eruption is a bright-red, and of an erysipelatous appearance.

Dose.—Four globules three times a day.

Rhus toxicodendron, if the inflamed surface is covered with blisters. It may be given alternately with Belladonna, and in obstinate cases with Mercurius vivus.

Dose.—Four globules three times a day.

Arsenicum, if the skin is dry and parchment-like, and the eruption presents a dark appearance, with a tendency to become gangrenous. Vomiting of food, or acrid bilious matter, with offensive green discharges from the bowels; also where the scrotum is affected.

Dose.—Six globules twice a day.

Sulphur, where there is some constitutional predisposition to the disease, and for inactivity of the alimentary canal after the acute symptoms are passed.

Dose.—Six globules once a day.

DENTITION.

The two middle lower front teeth make their appearance generally when the child is about six months old. In three or four weeks afterwards, the middle incisors of the upper jaw come through the gums, then comes the two lateral incisors below, which are soon followed by the two lateral incisors above. In about two months after these, the first four jaw teeth are cut, two below and two above; and after another little respite, the two stomach teeth and the two eye-teeth show themselves; and finally, at the age of from two years to two and a half, the four back jaw-teeth, two above and two below, make their appearance, which completes the first dentition, consisting of twenty teeth.

Every child does not cut its teeth with so much regularity as is indicated above, for some deviate variously from the rule which governs the ma jority.

The process of teething gives rise to a variety of sympathetic affections in children, many of which cause great suffering, and some of them are attended with considerable danger.

In order to save the child as much suffering as possible, if it still nurse, the mother should ab stain from all stimulating and indigestible articles, as well as everything else which she knows from experience will cause her milk to disagree with the child. And if the child be weaned, let its diet be of the most mild and unirritating kind—allow no coffee, tea, or malt liquors—no candies or other confectionaries. On account of the known tendency to heat in the head, sore ears, &c., during dentition, it is better for the child to sleep without a night-cap. Some children pass through the whole process without the least sickness.

Before the teeth come through, the gums usually become broader, more angular, and frequently show the shape of the coming teeth; the veins running parallel with the teeth become enlarged, and look like little red strings. The mouth becomes hot, and the child seems uneasy, particularly at night; its face is alternately flushed and pale; puts its fingers in its mouth; frequently seizes the nipple, bites, and then jerks its head away; the gums swell and become painful; the child drivels at the mouth, and the bowels become loose. When there is much constitutional disturbance, the child leans its head on the nurse's shoulder, becomes feverish; the skin is hot, with burning in the palms of the hands; the head is hot, and the feet cold; nausea and vomiting, with rubbing of the nose and frequent cough at night, during sleep.

When the gums are swollen and inflamed, and if the above enumerated sympathetic and constitutional symptoms be present, and especially if watery vesicles form over the teeth, giving the gums a rounded and bluish appearance, there is no valid objection to lancing. To perform this very simple, but useful operation properly, a *gum lancet* should be used; place the instrument over the tooth, and cut *through* the gum, until the tooth is felt.

The operation of lancing the gums is but seldom called for, as, in a majority of instances, a little timely interference with one or more of the following medicines will remove all the unpleasant symptoms.

REMEDIES. *Aconite*, *Belladonna*, *Calcarea carbonica*, *Chamomilla*, *Cina*, *Coffea*, *Ignatia*, *Ipecacuanha*, *Mercurius vivus*, and *Sulphur*.

Aconite, when there is fever with much restlessness, sleeplessness and suffering of pain, as evinced by the child's crying and starting.

Dose.—Dissolve eight globules in a wineglassful of water, and give a teaspoonful every two or three hours, until the child is better.

Belladonna, when convulsions are caused by teething; the convulsion is followed by sound sleep, which continues for a long time, or until another paroxysm comes on. The child starts suddenly from its sleep, as if frightened, and looks around as if terrified, with an altered expression of countenance; the pupils of the eyes are enlarged, and the child stares at a particular spot; the whole body becomes stiff; with burning heat in the palms of the hands and on the temples.

Dose.—Six globules dissolved in three tablespoonsful of water, and a teaspoonful to be given every twenty or thirty minutes, according to the severity of the case, until relief is afforded.

Calcarea carbonica, when the process of dentition is retarded in children of light complexion, and inclined to be fat.

Dose.—Six globules dissolved in a teaspoonful of water twice a week, for several weeks in succession.

Chamomilla is particularly adapted to the various diseases of children generally, during the period of dentition, and especially when a child is very uneasy at night; tosses about; wants drink often; has spasmodic jerks and twitches of the limbs during sleep; starts from the slightest noise; general heat; redness of the one cheek, and of the eyes; moaning; groaning; agitation; short, quick, noisy respiration, and oppression of the chest; hacking cough; mouth dry and hot; diarrhœa, with watery, slimy, and greenish evacuations, worse at night.

Dose.—Four globules in a teaspoonful of water, three times a day.

Cina may be given to children who wet the bed at night, and grit their teeth during sleep and at other times; have hardness and distension of the abdomen; rub their nose, and have a dry cough, resembling hooping-cough.

Dose.—Dissolve eight globules in a wineglassful of water, and give a teaspoonful three times a day.

Coffea, when the child is very excitable; does not sleep; is sometimes fretful, and at other times too lively, with some fever.

Dose.—Three globules dissolved in a teaspoonful of water, night and morning.

Ignatia, when there is convulsive jerkings of single limbs; frequent flushes of heat, sometimes followed by perspiration; the child rouses from a light sleep with piercing cries, and trembles all over.

Dose.—Six globules dissolved in a wineglassful of water, and a teaspoonful to be given every one, two, or three hours, according to the urgency of the case.

Ipecacuanha is very useful in nausea, and vomiting with diarrhœa; the stools are mixed, and of different colors.

Dose.—Three globules every two or three hours, until relief is afforded.

Mercurius vivus, is applicable in cases of copious driveling, redness of the gums, and green evacuations from the bowels, with straining.

Dose.—Four globules dissolved in a teaspoonful of water three times a day.

Sulphur may be given when the stools are whitish, or hot and sour, and excoriate the nates.

Dose.—The same as directed for Ipecacuanha.

SPASMS, OR CONVULSIONS.

Children from the period of their birth, until they attain their fourth year, are exceedingly liable to suffer from this disease. Between the ages specified, the nervous system of a child is more susceptible to the action of morbific agents, as well as influences of every kind, than it is in after life; hence judicious surgeons do not perform operations on very young children, when it can be postponed to a later period. A knowledge of this fact should deter physicians from bleeding and blistering at such an early age; and experience teaches all who witness such things and wish to learn, that the constitution of a young child cannot bear such treatment, without being injured by it. The circulation of the blood, and every vitalizing process is carried forward with greater rapidity than at any subsequent time; and hence accidental and mechanical injuries, such as cuts, fractures, and the like, are repaired in shorter time than they can be in after life.

So long as this susceptible and excitable state continues, just so long will the liability to convulsions remain, and the danger of an attack will be proportionate to the degree of excitability. Another predisposing cause, is the tendency to such diseases inherited from parents. The children in large and crowded cities are also more disposed to have such diseases than children in the country, who are favored with a purer atmosphere, and enjoy greater opportunities of exercise.

Among the exciting causes may be enumerated, dentition, the fever attending eruptive diseases, repelled eruptions, worms, errors in diet, falls upon the head, and mental emotions.

When a child is attacked with convulsions, let those having charge of it endeavor to be calm, and first of all, try to ascertain the exciting cause, and then become acquainted with the mode of attack, as upon these, in many instances, mainly depend the certainty and success of the treatment. In a majority of cases, the convulsions of young children are not dangerous, unless they occur during the advanced stage of the diseases incidental to childhood.

For the purpose of giving temporary relief, the child's feet and legs may be placed in warm water, and after being kept there for five or ten minutes, wiped dry and wrapped in flannel—the child's head should be sponged with cold water, or have the cold water poured on it through the spout of a tea-pot, from a height of three feet. If the child be costive, or it be suspected that there are some irritating matters in the bowels, give an injection of warm water, or molasses and water. If the child have eaten something that has disagreed with its stomach, and there be retching and vomiting, put a large mustard poultice over the stomach. If the child be cutting teeth, and the gums over the teeth next due be swollen, lance them. If the convulsions are caused by a fall, after the spasms are relieved, give Arnica.

Dose.—Dissolve twelve globules in a wineglassful of water, and give half a teaspoonful every ten or fifteen minutes; at the same time, if any of the parts are bruised, they may be bathed with a solution of Arnica tincture in water, in the proportion of thirty drops of the tincture to half a pint of water.

REMEDIES. *Belladonna*, *Chamomilla*, *Cina*, *Coffea*, *Hyoscyamus*, *Ignatia*, *Ipecacuanha*, *Mercurius vivus*, *Opium*, and *Stramonium*.

But for the purpose of curing the spasms, and

preventing their return, we must administer one or more of the above named medicines successively, according to the symptoms. The most favorable time for giving the medicines, is just as the fit is going off; but when the paroxysm lasts a long time, or one succeeds another with rapidity, the medicine must be given immediately, without waiting for the fit to terminate. If the first dose produces no change, repeat it in ten minutes, but if the child improve after the first dose, give nothing more so long as the improvement continues; when the symptoms get worse, or another paroxysm comes on, repeat the same medicine. If the remedy first given does not remove the disease, select another according to the symptoms.

Belladonna, if the paroxysm terminate in a state of stupor, or the child wakes suddenly, as if from fright, with staring eyes, fixed look, and dilated pupils; bending backwards; rigidity and coldness of the whole body, with burning in the hands and forehead; involuntary passages of fæces and urine.

Dose.—Dissolve twelve globules in a wineglassful of water, and give a teaspoonful of the solution every ten or fifteen minutes, until relief is afforded.

Chamomilla, if there be convulsive jerkings of the arms and legs; twitchings of the eye-lids and muscles of the face, with involuntary movements of the head from side to side, followed by drowsiness, with the eyes half open, and loss of consciousness; redness of one cheek, and paleness of the other; moaning, and frequent desire for drink; great restlessness and excitability. If the Chamomilla be not sufficient alone, it may be given alternately with Belladonna.

Dose.—The same as directed for Belladonna.

Cina, in children who are subject to worms, and are in the habit of wetting the bed, with spasms in the chest, convulsive movements of the limbs; distension and hardness of the abdomen; itching in the nose and of the anus, with loose cough at night.

Dose.—Dissolve six globules in a wineglassful of water, and give of the solution a teaspoonful every one, two, or three hours.

Coffea, in weakly, nervous children, who are frequently attacked by convulsions without any apparent cause.

Dose.—The same as directed for Cina.

Hyoscyamus, when twitchings of the muscles of the face and frothing of the mouth are the prominent symptoms.

Dose.—Four globules dissolved in a teaspoonful of water, every twenty or thirty minutes.

Ignatia may be considered the principal remedy

in the treatment of convulsions of children, inasmuch as it is more generally applicable than any other medicine, especially in the onset of the disease, when the cause is unknown. It is applicable, when particular parts or limbs are convulsed, or when the flesh here and there is affected by spasms, with frequent heat; light slumber with violent starts, screams and trembling of the whole body; perspiration; in children that are subject to fits, when the fits return every day, or every second day, at about the same hour, and are followed by heat and perspiration. Chamomilla is often suitable after Ignatia.

Dose.—The same as directed for Cina.

Ipecacuanha, when the child is asthmatic, sick at the stomach, with retching and vomiting, and has diarrhœa, and stretches itself out before, during, or after the paroxysm.

Dose.—Dissolve six globules in a wineglassful of water, and give a teaspoonful of the solution every hour.

Mercurius vivus if worms be the cause; saliva runs out of the mouth; green, watery stools; hard and distended abdomen; eructations; the child's skin is hot and moist; great weakness and exhaustion after the fits.

Dose.—The same as directed for Ipecacuanha.

Opium, when there is much trembling over the

whole body, tossing of the arms and legs, loud screaming during the paroxysm; the child lies unconscious as if stunned; the abdomen is swollen; suppression of urine and fæces. This remedy is particularly applicable if the fit have been caused by nursing, after the mother had been frightened or fallen into a passion.

Dose.—Dissolve six globules in three tablespoonsful of water, and a teaspoonful every fifteen or thirty minutes.

Stramonium, if the convulsions arise from repelled eruptions, or occur during the fever of eruptive diseases, or in consequence of eruptions not coming out; attended with involuntary evacuations of fæces and urine; much groping about with the hands, and opening and shutting of the fingers.

Dose.—The same as directed for Hyoscyamus.

SUMMER COMPLAINT.

Cholera infantum, as this disease is technically called, is generally owing to improper diet, either on the part of the mother or child, atmospheric changes, improper clothing, teething, and want of fresh air.

In some instances the disease begins like a simple diarrhœa, and is then frequently ascribed to the teeth alone, and very improperly neglected.

In its more aggravated forms, it commences with vomiting; first of the food, and afterwards of mucus, or mere gagging with efforts to vomit. The child's flesh becomes soft; it loses its appetite; has fever with evening exacerbations; the eyes look languid, and when the child sleeps, are but half closed. The thirst for cold water becomes very urgent, and all drink is immediately rejected by the stomach. The head and abdomen are hot, while the extremities are cold. The evacuations from the bowels are very frequent, and assume various appearances. Sometimes consisting of a mere looseness, at other times they are greenish, or yellow and watery, or they may be slimy and tinged with blood. The most common color, however, is white; the odor is very peculiar, and sometimes exceedingly offensive. The food frequently passes off without being digested.

In bad cases, the skin on the forehead is tight and shiny; the eyes are sunken; the cheeks fall in; the nose is sharp; the lips are shriveled; and the emaciation is extreme, so much so that the skin on the extremities hang in folds.

During the season in which children are most liable to the disease, they should be kept cool and frequently taken into the fresh air. Small children in cities are very much benefited by riding them out two or three miles into the country late in the afternoon to get ice cream, and then return before dark. A ride on the water by steamboat late in the afternoon, in very warm weather, is also very serviceable. Never take them out in the morning for the sake of health, so as to be obliged to return in the middle of the day, when it is warmer than when you went out.

Give the child no tea, coffee, and nothing sour or highly seasoned, no unripe fruit, or pies made of it; neither ought the mother to indulge in any article which she knows from experience will cause her milk to disagree with the child. The diet should be of the simplest kind; if the child be still at the breast, it should take but little else, and the mother should live on beef, mutton, and ham, of animal food, and milk or cocoa, bread and butter, potatoes and other vegetables of the most unirritating kind. If the child be weaned, pay strict attention to its diet as above directed. Give it a portion of *smoked herring* two or three times a week, in the morning for breakfast.

REMEDIES. *Antimonium crudum*, *Arsenicum*, *Bryonia*, *Carbo vegetabilis*, *Dulcamara*, *Ipecacuanha*, *Mercurius vivus*, *Nux vomica*, and *Veratrum*.

Antimonium crudum, when the tongue is coated white or yellow; dryness of the mouth, with thirst; nausea with vomiting, or gagging and cough; distension of the abdomen, with flatu lency; offensive, slimy stools, and frequent passages of water.

Dose.—Three globules in a teaspoonful of water after every discharge from the bowels.

Arsenicum, if the child be very weak, pale, and emaciated; inflation of the abdomen; cold extremities; loss of appetite; nausea and vomiting; intense thirst; yellow and watery, white or *brownish*, offensive diarrhœa, which is worse after midnight, towards morning, and after eating or drinking

Dose.—Dissolve twelve globules in a wineglassful of water, and give a teaspoonful every four hours until better.

Bryonia, when the diarrhœa comes on in *hot* weather, and is accompanied by much thirst; vomiting of food; nausea and vomiting after eating; diarrhœa, with colic; the stools have a putrid smell, are white, or brownish and lumpy.

Dose.—Four globules in a teaspoonful of water every six hours until relief is obtained.

Carbo vegetabilis, if Bryonia afford but temporary relief, especially if the evacuations be very thin and offensive and are attended with burning and much pain.

Dose.—The same as directed for Bryonia.

Dulcamara, if the complaint return every time the weather gets cold, or takes place after drinking cold water while in a heat; burning thirst for cold water; diarrhœa of a greenish or brownish mucus—worse at night.

Dose.—Three globules in a teaspoonful of water, every four hours.

Ipecacuanha, if given in the commencement of the disease, will generally arrest its progress at once. The symptoms which indicate Ipecacuanha are chiefly nausea and vomiting of ingesta, or mucus and bile, attended with diarrhœa of fermented stools of white flocks or tinged with blood; coated tongue; dislike to all food, and raging thirst.

Dose.—The same as directed for Antimonium crudum.

Mercurius vivus, when the diarrhœa is worse before midnight, and is attended with colic, straining at stool, and perspiration; evacuations are scanty, greenish, sour, and attended with nausea and eructation.

Dose.—Six globules dissolved in four teaspoonfuls of water, and a teaspoonful to be given every three hours until better.

Nux vomica, if Ipecacuanha should not be efficacious in arresting the disease at the outset, give six globules of Nux vomica at night and another dose next morning.

Veratrum, when the weakness from the nausea and vomiting is so great as almost to cause fainting; great exhaustion, vomiting, and diarrhœa;

vomiting after swallowing the least liquid; the slightest movement excites vomiting; thirst for cold water; sensitiveness over the pit of the stomach; colic, with burning and cutting pains in the abdomen; loose, brownish, and blackish stools; and small unnoticed evacuations of liquid fæces.

Dose.—Three globules in a teaspoonful of water every four or six hours.

ATROPHY.

This affection is caused by the system not receiving a sufficient supply of nourishment from the food taken, for the subsistence and development of the organism. In other words, defective nutrition.

REMEDIES. *Calcarea carbonica*, *Arsenicum*, *Belladonna*, *China*, *Nux vomica*, *Rhus toxicodendron*, and *Sulphur*.

Calcarea carbonica, where there is emaciation; voracious appetite; enlargement of the glands of the mesentery; general weakness; clay-colored discharges from the bowels; softness of the flesh; and excitability of the nervous system.

Dose.—Six globules twice a day.

Arsenicum, dry and parchment-like skin; vomiting of food; frequent desire to drink, but little at a time; restlessness; sleep interrupted by starting and jerking; greenish or brown diarrhœa stools; passage of undigested food; night-sweats, &c.

Dose.—Six globules three times a day.

Belladonna, cough, with rattling of mucus in the throat; swelling of the glands of the neck; colic, with involuntary stools; suited to children with precocity of intellect.

Dose.—Six globules three times a day

China, emaciation; enlarged and tympanitic abdomen; night sweats; diarrhœa, with discharges of undigested food; pale face; disturbed sleep, &c.

Dose.—Six globules every four hours.

Nux vomica, yellow, bloated face; constipation of the bowels; large and distended abdomen, with much flatulency; and desire to eat, with vomiting of food.

Dose.—Six globules twice a day.

Rhus toxicodendron, great debility, with constant desire to lie down; hard and distended abdomen; slimy or bloody diarrhœa.

Dose.—Four globules three times a day.

Sulphur, in the majority of cases, where there is swelling of the inquinal glands; hard and distended abdomen; rattling of mucus in the throat; diarrhœa or constipation; complexion pale, with sunken eyes.

Dose.—Six globules twice a day.

RUPTURE, OR HERNIA.

Delicate children, with feeble constitutions, are most liable to this disease. If the child cries much, and appears to suffer a great deal of pain; if the skin becomes clammy, and yet the child screams without apparent cause, examine its groins, and if swellings are discovered in one or both of them, which were not there before, send for a homœopathic physician, and in the meantime administer one of the following remedies:

REMEDIES. *Nux vomica*, *Chamomilla*, *Aconite*, *Opium*, and *Sulphur*.

Nux vomica, where the tumor is not very tender or painful to the touch; the vomiting not violent; but where respiration is difficult and obstructed.

Dose.—Six globules every one or two hours, as the circumstances of the case may require.

Chamomilla will be serviceable, when the foregoing remedy has failed to relieve, and the child appears to be very fretful, and there is a relaxed state of the bowels; the discharges having an unhealthy appearance.

Dose.—Twelve globules dissolved in three tablespoonsful of water, and a teaspoonful to be given every two hours.

Aconite, where there is much fever, and there is

much inflammation of the part affected, with great sensibility to the least touch.

Dose.—Three globules every two hours until the violence of the symptoms abate.

Opium, when there is redness of the face; hard and distended abdomen.

Dose.—Three globules every hour until relief is obtained.

Sulphur, in many instances, will be found very useful, especially if the foregoing remedies have failed to produce much relief.

Dose.—Three globules night and morning.

Rupture of the navel is more common, but less painful, than the variety above mentioned. It can be successfully treated by placing an additional compress under the belly-band, containing in its folds some hard substance like a piece of sheet-lead or thick pasteboard.

SORENESS BEHIND THE EARS.

This affection is a species of excoriation, and should be treated in a similar manner. Apply water to the sores as seldom as possible; only washing them in warm water, without soap, for purposes of cleanliness, and mop them dry with a fine linen handkerchief, and powder them with wheaten starch finely pulverized, when there is too much moisture to be absorbed.

REMEDIES. *Calcarea carbonica*, *Graphites*, and *Sulphur.*

Calcarea carbonica, moist eruption behind the ears; painful to the touch; skin hot and dry, with violent itching.

Dose.—Six globules at night, for several nights in succession, and if no improvement take place, consult the following remedy

Graphites, where the eruption behind the ears scales off, causing violent itching; or where there is much moisture and soreness behind the ears.

Dose.—The same as directed for Calcarea carbonica.

Sulphur, scurfy eruption, consisting of small vesicles, accompanied with violent itching; lacerating pain in the ears, extending to the head.

Dose.—The same as directed for Calcarea carbonica.

RUNNING FROM THE EARS.

Young children are subject to abscesses, and running from the internal ears. These gatherings are generally preceded by a great deal of pain; the child screams and rolls its head about; starts out of its sleep; sometimes there is considerable fever; it involuntarily puts its hands to the ears, and will not lie down.

REMEDIES. *Chamomilla*, *Pulsatilla*, and *Sulphur.*

Chamomilla, lancinating pain in the ears, extending to the head; humming in the ears, as from the rushing of water; starting in sleep, with moaning and sudden cries.

Dose.—Four globules three times a day.

Pulsatilla, lancinating or darting pains through the ears, with heat, redness and swelling of the ears, or discharge of pus from the ears.

Dose.—Dissolve twelve globules in four tablespoonsful of water, and give a teaspoonful every two or three hours.

Sulphur, lancinating pain in the ears, extending to the head, or where the discharge of matter has already taken place.

Dose.—Six globules night and morning until better.

Pulsatilla is also applicable, after the running is established.

HORDEOLUM; OR STYE.

This is an inflammatory action of one of the glands in the margin of the eye-lid, of the nature of a boil, and mostly makes its appearance near the inner angle of the eye.

REMEDIES. *Pulsatilla*, *Aurum metalicum*, *Staphysagria*, *Arsenicum*, and *Sulphur*.

Pulsatilla is considered almost specific in this disease, as it mostly disappears after taking a few doses of it.

Dose.—Six globules three times a day.

Aurum metalicum, if the eyelids are red and

swollen, with obstruction and ulceration of the nostrils.

Dose.—Six globules night and morning.

Staphysagria, if they are of frequent recurrence, and leave a tendency to fresh inflammation, or if indurations and hardness of the eyelid remain.

Dose.—Six globules night and morning.

Arsenicum, scrofulous inflammation of the eyes, with odematous swelling of the lids; dryness of the margin of the lids.

Dose.—Six globules night and morning.

Sulphur, itching and inflammation of the eyelids; swelling of the lids, with pimples on them, and dryness.

Dose.—Six globules night and morning.

NOCTURNAL URINATION.

Constant "wetting the bed," in a majority of instances, is the result of disease, although in a few cases it may be owing to the indulgence in filthy habits. Whipping is a remedy that is frequently applied, but I never knew it to cure a single case.

Remedies. *Sepia*, *Silicea*, and *Cina*.

Sepia, continual desire to urinate; pressure on the bladder, with frequent discharges of urine; spasm of the neck of the bladder.

Dose.—Three globules for several nights in succession, and if no improvement take place consult the next remedy.

Silicea, micturition every night; desire to urinate, with pressure upon the bladder; yellow sediment like sand in the urine.

Dose.—Six globules for several nights in succession, to be given previous to going to bed.

Cina, if there is suspicion that worms are the cause, and there is involuntary emission of urine, which becomes turbid immediately after being passed.

Dose.—The same as directed for Silicea.

PROLAPSUS ANI.

The descent of the rectum, or the "body coming down," as it is termed in domestic language, is generally consequent upon some other disease. It is apt to follow upon long continued diarrhœa, or an acute attack of dysentery; protracted costiveness also may give rise to it, or it may depend on a state of relaxation of the system merely.

When the bowel is protruded, it can easily be reduced, by laying the child across the lap, and making pressure on the protruded part with a piece of fine linen cloth, anointed with fresh lard.

When it is but an attendant upon another dis

ease, of course that disease must be removed before the prolapsus can be cured. But when it stands out as a disease by itself, the following remedies will frequently cure it:

REMEDIES. *Ignatia*, *Nux vomica*, *Bryonia*, *Podophyllum pelt.*

Ignatia, desire for stool, with protrusion of the rectum; sharp pain in the rectum after stool; violent itching of the anus.

Dose.—Three globules three times a day until better.

Nux vomica, constipation, as if from contraction and constriction of the bowels of infants, especially from the use of coffee; frequent and ineffectual urging to stool.

Dose.—Four globules night and morning until better.

Bryonia, constipation; stool hard and dry, or, as if burnt, with protrusion of the rectum; long, lasting burning at the rectum after stool.

Dose.—The same as given for Nux vomica.

Podophyllum pelt. for the same symptoms, and to be given in the same way as directed for Ignatia.

WEANING.

As a general rule, children should be weaned when they are about eighteen months old.

If the mother is weakly, the supply of milk

begins to diminish in quantity, and deteriorate in quality, or the menses reappear, the child may be weaned at an earlier period.

The progressive development of a child's teeth may be taken as a sign, that the mother's milk may be dispensed with, and that its digestive organs are capable of managing more substantial food.

But a child ought not to be weaned while it is suffering very much from the irritation of teething, or other infantile diseases, unless there are considerations on the part of the mother which render it necessary.

As soon as the teeth begin to make their appearance, a child ought to be gradually accustomed to taking other kinds of nourishment; so that, by the time its jaw teeth come through, it may be able to eat a portion of animal as well as vegetable food. Let it have what is going at table besides its bread and milk, which should be the stand-by.

There is nothing gained to a healthy child by nursing through the second summer, the say-so of our grandmothers to the contrary notwithstanding. The most suitable seasons of the year for weaning are, March or April, in the spring, and October or November, in the fall.

After the process of weaning is decided upon,

be not deceived by the plausibility of the *theory* of doing it gradually, nor of keeping the breast from the child through the day, and of giving it to it through the night; as such a course not only prolongs the sufferings of the child, but also renders the milk unfit for the stomach. Nothing ought to induce a mother, except in case of sickness, to give her infant into the hands of another person, however competent she may be to perform the office for a child of her own, for the purpose of weaning. Neither ought a mother to absent herself from home, during the trying period; if she really love her offspring, let her extend her sympathy while she maintains sufficient firmness to do what is best for the child. It is grieved at her absence, besides losing its favorite nourishment; and then is doomed to disappointment on her return, which is almost as painful as the first privation.

The best and easiest method of weaning a child, is to take it to bed as usual, and in nothing depart from the common routine of management, except to withhold the breast. Once denied, let not the child have it again; and in forty-eight hours the whole process, so far as the child is concerned, will be completed. Give the child the food it is accustomed to, and do not pamper its stomach with candies and other sweetmeats.

After weaning, the child's diet should be simple,

but sufficiently nourishing; as intimated above, bread and milk should be the staple food, but the the farinaceous articles; such as arrow-root, tapioca, &c., or mashed potatoes, bread and butter, and occasionally a little beef, mutton, chicken, or good ham, may be allowed.

After the child is taken from the breast, let the mother abstain from salted articles, to prevent thirst; and as far as she can from fluid nourishment of every sort, in order to diminish the secretion of milk; eat only the driest kind of food, drink nothing but water and that in small quantities. If the breasts be painfully distended with milk, rub them with hot lard, and wrap them in raw cotton. In order to get rid of the distension, it is generally necessary to have the breasts drawn; but let this be done only so far as it is necessary to give present relief, and as seldom as possible; increasing the interval between each time of drawing, so as not to encourage the secretion of more milk.

REMEDIES. *Pulsatilla*, *Rhus toxicodendron*, *Bryonia*, and *Belladonna*.

Pulsatilla will be found one of the most efficient remedies to stop the secretion of the milk, especially where there is pressure and swelling of the breasts.

Dose.—Twelve globules dissolved in a wineglassful of water, and a teaspoonful taken three times day.

Rhus toxicodendron may be used with much be nefit, where there is soreness and swelling of the breasts brought on by cold.

Dose.—The same as directed for Pulsatilla.

Bryonia, if the breasts are hard, and too full of milk, with tensive and shooting pain, or burning heat.

Dose.—Four globules three times a day.

Belladonna, erysipelatous inflammation of the breasts, particularly from weaning; swelling and induration of the breasts, or where there is too great a secretion of milk.

Dose.—The same as directed for Pulsatilla.

LEUCORRHŒA OF CHILDREN.

Little girls, from a little neglect and some other incidental causes, are liable to a discharge of whitish mucus from the vagina, somewhat similar to the leucorrhœa of adults. Frequent ablutions with luke-warm water will generally remove it in a short time; but if it should not, give six globules of Calcarea carbonica, two nights in succession, and continue the washings.

PART III.

GENERAL DISEASES.

GENERAL DISEASES.

CATARRH; OR COLD IN THE HEAD.

THIS disease consists of a mild degree of inflammation of the mucous membrane lining the larynx and nostrils, and sometimes extends as far as the bronchial ramifications, and is mostly caused by sudden exposure, from heat to cold. The most prominent symptoms of this disease are the following: slight febrile excitement; want of appetite; sneezing; obstruction of the nose; pain in the head, back, and extremities, followed by discharge of mucus from the nose, which soon becomes watery; and it is always attended, more or less, with slight wheezing and difficult respiration.

REMEDIES. *Aconite*, *Mercurius vivus*, *Nux vomica*, *Chamomilla*, *Dulcamara*, *Pulsatilla*, *Rhus toxicodendron*, and *Arsenicum*.

Aconite will be found useful in the commencement of the disease, if there is any fever; violent sneezing; scraping sensation in the throat; violent thirst; short dry cough, with short and hurried respiration.

Dose.—Three globules every one or two hours, until the inflammatory symptoms are subdued, after which another remedy may be required.

Mercurius vivus will be of great service, if there is continual sneezing and swelling of the whole nose, and discharge of profuse fluent coryza; profuse perspiration at night; especially if the attack was brought about by exposure to a raw atmosphere.

Dose.—Six globules three times a day until better, or the symptoms require another remedy.

Nux vomica, if there is dryness of the mouth and throat; heat of the face; stoppage of the nose at night, and discharge during the day; continual heat in the nose; dullness of the head; aversion to food and drinks; oppression of the chest, and constipation.

Dose.—The same as directed for Aconite.

Chamomilla, if the attack has been caused by sudden changes from heat to cold, or check of perspiration; obstruction of the nose, with discharge of mucus; throbbing headache; pain in the throat, as from a plug, when swallowing.

Dose.—Three globules every four hours.

Dulcamara, if there is oppression of the chest, with short hacking cough; dry coryza, with dullness of the head; and sneezing, and the least exposure renews the attack.

Dose.—Three globules three times a day.

Pulsatilla, if there is loss of smell, or green fetid discharge from the nose; scraping and dryness in the throat; cough, with expectoration of yellow mucus.

Dose.—The same as directed for Chamomilla.

Rhus toxicodendron, stoppage of the nose; complete loss of appetite; especially if the attack has been caused by getting wet.

Dose.—The same as directed for Chamomilla.

Arsenicum, if the discharge from the nose is very acrid and corrosive; soreness of the nostrils and burning of the nose.

Dose.—Four globules three times a day.

SIMPLE FEVER, INFLAMMATORY FEVER.

This variety of fever is characterized by violent heat; burning; hot and dry skin; full pulse, which is mostly hard and tight; tongue dry and bright-red, and frequently white-coated; great thirst; urine bright-red and burning; great restlessness; violent headache and sleeplessness.

REMEDIES. *Aconite*, *Belladonna*, *Chamomilla*, *Mercurius vivus*, and *Bryonia*.

Aconite is especially indicated, where there is hot, dry skin; great thirst; congestion to the head or chest; redness of the cheeks; headache, and nightly delirium; shortness of breath, with dry hacking cough; urine scanty, and highly colored.

Dose.—Eight globules dissolved in a tumbler half-full of water and a teaspoonful to be given every half, one, two, or three hours according to the violence of the symptoms.

Belladonna, where there are symptoms of con gestion toward the brain; face red and puffed, with burning heat; pulse full and quick; violent thirst and delirium; eyes prominent and congested; or where there is delirium.

Dose.—The same as directed for Aconite.

Chamomilla, especially if the attack has been brought on by anger, and there is throbbing headache; excessive heat, with violent thirst; redness of the cheeks, with delirium; palpitation of the heart, and great irritability of temper.

Dose.—Three globules every hour until better, or the symptoms indicate another remedy.

Mercurius vivus, if there is violent thirst; continual coldness of the hands and feet; pulse accelerated and irregular; disposition to profuse sweat; constant desire for cold water.

Dose.—Six globules every three or four hours until better.

Bryonia, dry, burning heat, alternating with chills; violent thirst; great excitement of the vascular system, or if there is congestion of the chest; headache, as if the contents would issue through the forehead; also, if it is accompanied with gastric disturbance.

Dose.—Three globules in a teaspoonful of water every three hours.

BRAIN FEVER.

Brain fever is distinguished from simple fever by constant drowsiness or delirium; fullness and redness of the face and eyes; congestion of blood to the brain; violent beating of the carotid and temporal arteries; dullness of vision; the eyes congested; pupils either dilated or contracted; headache, with constant giddiness; restlessness, with constant tossing about; cannot bear the least light, which causes the patient to scream and become discontented; eyes convulsed and fixed; pupils immoveable.

REMEDIES. *Aconite, Belladonna, Bryonia, Hyoscyamus, Opium, Stramonium,* and *Cuprum aceticum.*

Aconite, in the commencement of the disease, where there is hot and dry skin; pulse full and quick; sleeplessness, with continual tossing about; fullness and heaviness in the brain, as if it would press through the forehead, with throbbing in the temples.

Dose.—Six globules dissolved in a wineglassful of water, and a teaspoonful of the solution every hour until better.

Belladonna, if there is much heat and dullness in the head; face red and bloated; strong, quick, and full pulse; eyes congested and sparkling, with great sensibility and aversion to light; wild look from the eyes; throbbing of the arteries of the head and neck.

Dose.—The same as directed for Aconite.

Bryonia, if there is great weight in the head; delirious talk at night during sleep; bloatedness of the face; congestion of blood to the head; continual inclination to sleep; sleep, with twitchings of the muscles of the face.

Dose.—Six globules in a teaspoonful of water, every two or three hours, as the circumstances of the case may require.

Hyoscyamus, if there is loss of consciousness; eyes staring and distorted; face red and bloated; burning and dryness of the tongue; foam at the mouth; grasping at flocks; small, weak, irregular pulse; picking of the bed-clothes with the fingers.

Dose.—Four globules every two hours until better.

Opium, where there is a constant disposition to sleep; starts in sleep; sleep restless and full of moaning; delirium; hot skin; congestion of blood to the head; eyes staring and glistening; the pupils insensible to light; face pale and sunken.

Dose.—Six globules in a teaspoonful of water every hour until better.

Stramonium, delirium; stupefaction of the senses; starting and jerking in the limbs; swelling and redness of the eyes and face; eyes sparkling and staring; redness of the whites of the eyes; strong full pulse, with moisture of the skin.

Dose.—The same as directed for Belladonna.

Cuprum aceticum, starting during sleep; convulsive movements of the limbs; feverish heat; pulse hard and contracted; painful throbbing of the temporal arteries; the eyes are sunken and staring.

Dose.—Give three globules every two or three hours until better.

INFANTILE REMITTENT FEVER.

The form of remittent fever which occurs in infants and children, is generally attended by morbid irritability or inflammation, and may terminate in ulceration of the lining membrane of the whole alimentary canal. It is commonly caused by undue exposure to cold; the irritation of teething; the use of improper and indigestible articles of diet; rich cake, nuts, sweet-meats, &c.

This disease ismostly preceded by languor; irritable mood; nausea and qualmishness; want of appetite; thirst; dry skin; difficult and hurried breathing; accelerated pulse; inflated abdomen; vomiting of food; tongue moist and coated, the margin presenting a very red appearance; constipation or diarrhœa, with fœtid discharges, mixed with mucus or blood: there is generally great restlessness and thirst. There is often coolness of the hands and feet, whilst the head and body are preternaturally hot, with drowsiness through the day; followed by general development of heat in the evening, with increase of fever and delirium through the night.

REMEDIES. *Ipecacuanha*, *Pulsatilla*, *China*, *Nux vomica*, *Belladonna*, *Mercurius*, *Bryonia*, *Chamomilla*, and *Sulphur*.

Ipecacuanha, if the attack was brought on by overfeeding, or indigestible food; dry heat of skin; thirst; restlessness; impeded breathing; foul coated tongue; nausea and vomiting.

Dose.—Three globules every two or three hours.

Pulsatilla, relaxation of the bowels; white or bilious stools, with fullness and griping in the bowels; or if the attack was brought on by rich food, fat pork, &c.

Dose.—Six globules three times a day.

China, if the abdomen remain tense or tympanitic, and the vomiting has subsided, and there is much weakness.

Dose.—Six globules three times a day.

Nux vomica, if there is constipation, with frequent urging to stool; abdomen painful; foul tongue; nausea and disgust for food; gulping up of bitter or sour fluid; stomach sensitive to pressure; cutting in the abdomen.

Dose.—The same as directed for Pulsatilla

Belladonna, if there are inflammatory symptoms; great heat of the head; fullness of the pulse; heat of the abdomen, with tenderness upon pressure; tongue coated in the centre, white or yellow, with red edges.

Dose.—Four globules every four hours.

Mercurius vivus, after Belladonna, when the following symptoms present themselves: abdomen tender upon pressure, or tenesmus with diarrhœa; coated tongue; quick pulse, and aversion to drinks.

Dose.—Four globules three times a day.

Bryonia, if there is heaviness of the head, with a dull feeling; excited pulse; coated tongue, or other signs of gastric disturbance; constipation; hurried respiration; tenderness of the abdomen, and drowsiness.

Dose.—The same as directed for Pulsatilla.

Chamomilla, if there are bilious vomitings or diarrhœa; burning heat of the skin; yellow coated tongue; agitation; quick pulse, and jerking in the limbs.

Dose.—The same as Pulsatilla.

Sulphur, flushes of heat, with alternate paleness of the face; dry skin; hurried breathing; oppression of the chest, with palpitation of the heart; hard or loose stools.

Dose.—Six globules night and morning.

RACHITIS; OR RICKETS.

This disease usually shows itself in children as early as one or two years of age, and is distinguished by the slow and imperfect acquisition of the power of standing and walking; abnormal development of the head; prominence of the forehead; enlargement of the bones about the joints; projection of the sternum; flattening of the ribs; curvature of the spine; tumefaction of the abdomen, with waddling gait; predisposition to diarrhœa, accompanied with slow fever, difficulty of breathing, and general emaciation. Children of a scrofulous diathesis are more liable to this disease than others. With the growth and development of the body, this disease sometimes disappears of itself.

REMEDIES. *Belladonna*, *Mercurius*, *Sulphur*, *Calcarea carbonica*, *Silicea*, *Phosphoric acid*, *Nitric acid*, and *Pulsatilla*.

Belladonna, where there is hardness and distension of the abdomen, as is always the case in curvature of the bones, especially of the spine, with unsteady staggering gait; looseness of the muscles, and fullness of the countenance.

Dose.—Six globules night and morning.

Mercurius, where there is heaviness of the limbs; great weakness of the knees; cracking of the joints; pain in all of the bones of the head; clay-colored face; enlargement of the abdomen; and especially in those disposed to glandular enlargements.

Dose.—Six globules night and morning.

Sulphur is one of the most appropriate remedies in all stages of this disease; especially where there is curvature of the spine; enlargement of the bones of the head, or bones of the wrist; muscles thin and flaccid; stools irregular; paleness of the face, with violent pressure in the head.

Dose.—Six globules twice a day.

Calcarea carbonica, if the fontanelles are open too long; softness of the ends of the long bones; and where the spine appears too weak to carry the weight of the body, owing to a deficiency of calcareous deposit in the bones.

Dose.—Dissolve twelve globules in half a tumbler of water, and of the solution give a teaspoonful three times a day.

Silicea, in diseases of the bones in general, especially in children, with enlarged head and slowly closing fontanelles; or where there is muscular weakness, with difficulty of learning to walk hot distended abdomen; aching pain in the sternum; violent pain in the small of the back, with swelling and curvature of the spine.

Dose.—The same as directed for Calcarea.

Phosphoric acid, swelling of the joints, evil consequences of too rapid growth, inflammation of the bones, and languor of the whole body.

Dose.—Four globules twice a day.

Nitric acid, lancinating pains in the limbs; burning in the joints, with weakness as if paralyzed; emaciation; heaviness; pain in the small of the back, as if from stiffness.

Dose.—Three globules three times a day.

Pulsatilla, curvature of the lower portion of the spine; the heads of the bones large and prominent; fontanelles widely open; but little hair on the head; staring looks; muscles thin and flabby; abdomen large and flaccid.

Dose.—Six globules twice a day.

BOLD HIVES, NETTLE RASH; OR URTICARIA.

This is a very common eruptive disease of children, and is known by large, red, and diffused patches, or wheals of various sizes and irregular shapes, resembling the stings of nettles; or in streaks. The elevations generally are of a pale, but occasionally of a bright red color, white in the centre. Sometimes the eruption is paler than the surrounding skin. It is accompanied with burning and troublesome itching, especially when the patient gets warm in bed, causing continual scratching, and is mostly preceded by gastric disturbance: such as nausea and vomiting, restlessness, languor, thirst, want of appetite, and coated tongue, with more or less febrile excitement.

After the eruption has made its appearance, the gastric disturbance and febrile excitement gradually disappear, and nothing is left but the itching caused by the eruption.

This disease is frequently brought on by errors in diet, indigestion, or a faulty state of the skin and its secretion. In those who have a constitutional predisposition to the disease, it may be excited by a particular article of food, as shell-fish, almonds, honey, mushrooms, cucumbers, and acid fruits.

REMEDIES. *Aconite*, *Dulcamara*, *Pulsatilla*, *Rhus toxicodendron*, *Bryonia*, *Belladonna*, *Hepar sulphur*, *Arsenicum*, *Calcarea carbonica*, *Nux vomica*, *Sulphur*, and *Urtica urens.*

Aconite, if with the eruption there is much fever; hard, accelerated pulse; dry and hot skin; much thirst; coated tongue, with restlessness and anxiety

Dose.—Four globules every two or three hours, according to the state of the case.

Dulcamara, if the patient has been exposed to damp and wet weather; has fever; bitter taste in the mouth; diarrhœa, and coated tongue, with itching and burning after scratching.

Dose.—Four globules every four hours.

Pulsatilla, if the attack has been brought on by fat or indigestible food; or is accompanied with looseness of the bowels. Pulsatilla is particularly adapted to persons of an even temperament and quiet disposition, and especially females and children.

Dose.—Four globules three times a day.

Rhus toxicodendron is adapted to many cases of this disorder, especially where it arises from a peculiarity of the constitution; or if the eruption is caused by some particular kind of food, and scratching increases the irritation.

Dose.—Six globules twice a day.

Bryonia, if the eruption has been suddenly suppressed, and is attended with difficulty of breathing and oppression of the chest.

Dose.—Four globules three times a day.

Belladonna, if with the eruption there is congestion to the head, with red face, giddiness and headache.

Dose.—Three globules four times a day.

Hepar sulphur will be useful if the eruption is attended with catarrhal symptoms, as cold in the head, with coryza, affecting only one side.

Dose.—Six globules night and morning.

Nux vomica, if the eruption is excited by the use of stimulants; or where there is much gastric derangement, constipation, indigestion, &c.

Dose.—Six globules night and morning.

Sulphur, if the disease has been suppressed, will be found very serviceable in restoring the eruption to the surface.

Dose.—Four globules three times a day until the eruption is brought out again.

Urtica urens is found very useful in many cases, if the eruption has a pale and hard appearance, and causes a great deal of scratching.

Dose.—Six globules every two or three hours.

RINGWORM; OR HERPES CIRCINNATUS.

This is a common affection, especially in children, and consists of an eruption of small circular vesicles of a red appearance (the skin in the internal portion of the ring retaining the natural color) at first, but soon becomes rough, and of a brownish hue, and finally scales off as the eruption dies away.

This disease mostly appears on the face, neck, arms, and shoulders, and may continue for two or three weeks, and even a greater length of time.

REMEDIES. *Sepia*, *Rhus toxicodendron*, *Sulphur*, *Hepar sulphur*, and *Calcarea carbonica.*

Sepia will, in most cases, remove this disease, and will generally prevent the formation of new rings.

Dose.—Six globules twice a day.

Rhus toxicodendron, burning in the face as if ulcerated; skin hot, with the feeling as if there was an eruption there; crusty eruption in the face.

Dose.—Four globules three times a day.

Sulphur will be useful where there is a general predisposition to this affection.

Dose.—Six globules every night.

Hepar sulphur may be used if matter is formed.

Dose.—Six globules twice a day.

Calcarea carbonica, in obstinate cases, and in persons of a scrofulous diathesis.

Dose.—Six globules every night.

PRICKLY HEAT; OR HEAT SPOTS.

Infants and children are often attacked in warm weather with an eruption of small vesicles, about the size of a pin's head, which sometimes fill with a thin, watery fluid; at other times they are red and inflamed, and attended with more or less fever, which makes the child very irritable, and causes it continually to scratch the parts affected. The duration of this disease is very uncertain, and apt to disappear in cool weather, and return again when it becomes warm.

If it does not interfere too much with the child's comfort, better let it alone. In aggravated cases we may resort to one of the following

REMEDIES. *Aconite*, *Chamomilla*, *Bryonia*, *Rhus toxicodendron*, and *Sulphur*.

Aconite, if the eruption is accompanied with much fever, dry, hot skin, and restlessness.

Dose.—Four globules three times a day.

Chamomilla, if Aconite is not sufficient, and there is still great restlessness.

Dose.—The same as given of Aconite.

Bryonia, if the eruption is suppressed, accompanied with much restlessness, and the patient is excited and cannot bear to be moved.

Dose.—Four globules every three hours.

Sulphur will mostly relieve a tendency to this affection, or if the eruption manifests a disposition to spread.

Dose.—Six globules every night.

SCARLET RASH.

This disease which appears to be so similar to scarlet fever, presents some striking differences. It attacks persons of all ages, and the efflorescence consists of red spots or patches, which at times have a purplish or dark red tinge, and leaves no white mark from slight pressure with the finger. The patches are dotted, and thickly covered with red pimples or granules, which are a little raised above the surface, and may be distinctly seen and felt. The eruption is not confined to any particular part, but prefers those portions which are covered, especially about the joints.

Neither the eruption nor the fever are so well defined in their course, nor regular in the time of their disappearance, as are most other eruptive fevers. When the external manifestations of the disease disappear prematurely, disease of the brain, throat, &c., may follow, and involve the patient in great danger. The eruption may be very extensive, and still the attack not dangerous; or the eruption may be but trifling, and yet the disease be very dangerous. One attack does not exonerate a person from future liability. The premonitory symptoms of this disease are: chilliness followed by fever, dull feeling in the head, usually attended with catarrhal symptoms, and some derangement of stomach. The eruptions first appear in the face, then on the neck, back and chest, and afterward on the extremities. The bowels are generally costive, urine dark-colored and scanty, mouth dry and hot, throat sore, with thirst and restlessness.

REMEDIES. *Aconite*, *Belladonna*, *Ipecacuanha*, *Coffea*, *Pulsatilla*, *Bryonia*, *Dulcamara*, *Calcarea carbonica*, and *Stramonium.*

Aconite is generally considered specific for this disease, where it is not complicated with any other disease; especially if there is much fever, with full pulse, pale face, slight chills, drowsiness, oppression of the chest, &c.

Dose.—Six globules every two hours until the fever abates.

Belladonna, where there is cerebral disturbance, as congestion to the brain; or if the disease is complicated with scarlatina, sore throat, &c.

Dose.—Six globules every two hours.

Ipecacuanha may be useful if there is little fever, and the eruption is slow in making its appearance; or if there is nausea, vomiting, diarrhœa and restlessness.

Dose.—Six globules every two hours.

Coffea, where there are excessive pains, with great restlessness and anxiety.

Dose.—Six globules every hour.

Pulsatilla may be used if the disease is accompanied with acidity of the stomach, nausea, vomiting, or diarrhœa.

Dose.—Four globules every two hours.

Bryonia, if there are symptoms of internal congestion, with oppression and hurried or difficult breathing.

Dose.—Six globules every two hours.

Dulcamara, if accompanied with rheumatic pains in the limbs, or where the glands are swollen, and the throat but slightly affected.

Dose.—Four globules every three hours.

Calcarea carbonica, will be serviceable, where there is swelling of the glands, with inability to swallow, and ill humor.

Dose.—Six globules every three or four hours.

Stramonium, where there is stupor, with involuntary discharges of fæces and urine, &c.

Dose.—Six globules every hour.

SCARLATINA; OR SCARLET FEVER.

The simplest form of scarlet fever; is characterized by fever with an accelerated pulse, pain in the throat, with swelling, and after one or two days, a breaking out of scarlet spots, similar in color to the shell of a boiled lobster, diminishing in color as they approach the neighboring skin. At times it extends over the whole body, with a uniform redness. The eruption is smooth, and if pressed upon by the finger a white imprint remains, which disappears almost immediately after the pressure is discontinued. The eruptive stage terminates in from five to seven days, when the epidermis begins to peel off about the fingers, and in patches on other parts. The eruptive fever of simple scarlatina varies both in intensity and duration—at times it is very slight, at others more violent; the premonitory symptoms are generally a sense of weakness, indisposition, nausea and vomiting; then chilliness followed by heat, with pain in the throat, and headache. On the second day the eruption makes its appearance; first on the face and neck, then the chest, and gradually extends itself over the whole body. The parts on which the eruption first makes its appearance are generally those from which it first begins to disappear.

Scarlet fever is distinguished from measles, by not having the catarrhal symptoms which usually attends the latter disease: such as redness of the eyes, coryza, coughing, sneezing, &c., which generally decline as the eruption advances; while in scarlet fever, the appearance of the eruption affords no mitigation of the fever, sore throat, &c

The disease is divided into three stages. The first stage is characterized by fever, sore throat, greatly accelerated pulse, and frequently delirium.

The second stage begins with the eruption, continues four or five days, and ends with the decline of fever and the disappearance of the eruption. It is during this stage that the brain, throat, &c., are most liable to become dangerously involved in the disease.

It is in the third stage of the disease, extending from the seventh or eighth day to the third week—the stage of disquamation—that the sequalæ are most likely to make their appearance. The most common of which are abscesses, disease of the heart, and dropsical effusions.

REMEDIES. *Aconite*, *Belladonna*, *Rhus toxicodendron*, *Opium*, *Ipecacuanha*, *Pulsatilla*, *Mercurius vivus*, *Arsenicum*, *Calcarea carbonica*, *Phosphorus*, *Cuprum aceticum*, *Tartar emetic*, and *Nitric acid.*

Aconite will be useful in the very commencement of the disease, especially if there is much febrile excitement.

Dose.—Six globules every three hours until the fever is ameliorated.

If the eruption is slow about making its appearance, Bryonia or Sulphur may be given with advantage, alternately with Aconite, every two or three hours.

Belladonna, in the treatment of true scarlatina, either during the forming stage of the disease, or when it is more fully developed, may be considered one of our most important remedies. It is indicated by delirium, headache, sore throat, fever, &c.

Dose.—The same as Aconite.

Rhus toxicodendron is also important in the sore throat, aching pains, and itching of the skin.

Dose.—The same as Belladonna.

Opium may be used with benefit, if there is burning heat, stupefaction, tossing about, with vomiting, constipation, or convulsions.

Dose.—Four globules every one, two, or three hours, according to the symptoms.

Ipecacuanha, if there is an increase of fever toward evening, with sleeplessness, loss of appetite, nausea, vomiting, irritable mood, and moaning; should this remedy not relieve, it may be followed by Pulsatilla.

Dose.—Four globules every two hours.

Mercurius vivus, when Belladonna and Rhus have been insufficient, and there is the appearance of ulceration about the mouth and throat, with increased secretion of mucus, accompanied with swelling of the throat and tonsils.

Dose.—Six globules every three hours.

Arsenicum, should ulceration have already taken place, and the ulcers assume a livid appearance at the edges, with offensive odor, great loss of strength, thirst, restlessness, and diarrhœa.

Dose.—Six globules every three hours.

Calcarea carbonica, when the glands are much swollen, great dryness of the mouth and throat, swelling of the tonsils, and constriction of the throat.

Dose.—Six globules every three or four hours.

Phosphorus, when there is repercussion of the eruption, it will aid in restoring it; also where there is swelling of the tonsils, rawness, burning, and soreness in the posterior part of the throat.

Dose.—Six globules every two or three hours.

Cuprum aceticum, if upon repercussion of the eruption there should be symptoms of metastasis to the brain, paleness of the face, gagging, convulsions, jerking of the limbs, pains in the abdomen, &c.

Dose.—Dissolve twelve globules in half a tumbler of water, and of this solution give a teaspoonful every fifteen or twenty minutes, according to circumstances, until relief is obtained.

Tartar emetic may be given in the first stage, if the eruption is preceded by convulsions, cold sweat, and difficulty of breathing; or if it is attended with vomiting.

Dose.—The same as directed for Cuprum aceticum.

Nitric acid, if the disease should assume a malignant form, with ulceration of the throat.

Dose.—Six globules every four hours.

MEASLES; OR RUBEOLA.

This well known disease generally prevails as an epidemic once in six or seven years. It is communicated by contagion, and always makes its appearance with symptoms of catarrh, with dry cough, hoarseness, oppression of the chest, pain in the throat, sneezing, and acrid discharges from the nose, watery discharge from the eyes, headache, and sometimes nausea and vomiting.

The above symptoms, accompanied with more or less fever, usually precede the eruption from three to five days.

The eruption appears first on the face and neck, and then extends itself gradually over the rest of the body and limbs. It consists of small, red spots, resembling flea-bites, frequently arranged in semilunar lines, or small irregular arcs. In about four days after its appearance the eruption begins to turn pale, and disappears about the sixth day, with a bran-like exfoliation of the external skin.

REMEDIES. *Aconite*, *Belladonna*, *Bryonia*, *Mercurius*, *Arsenicum*, *Pulsatilla*, *Ipecacuanha*, *Sulphur*, *Phosphorus*, and *Dulcamara*.

Aconite is one of the most reliable remedies in

this disease, and will frequently shorten its course where there is fever; dry, hot skin; heat in the head; giddiness; redness of the eyes, and dread of light.

Dose.—Six globules every four hours.

Belladonna, if the throat becomes sore, with fever, headache, and delirium; difficult deglutition; spasmodic cough, with rattling in the throat; or if there is congestion toward the brain.

Dose.—Four globules every two or three hours.

Bryonia, if the eruption is not fully developed; difficulty of breathing, with stiches in the chest and dry cough.

Dose.—Six globules every two hours.

Mercurius, when the glands of the throat are much swollen, or violent sore throat, with difficulty of swallowing.

Dose.—Four globules every three hours.

Arsenicum, if there is dry, burning heat of the skin, accompanied with much thirst, and great prostration of strength.

Dose.—Four globules every two hours.

Pulsatilla, if given at the beginning of the disease, will be found almost specific for the catarrhal symptoms, and where the eruption is slow in making its appearance.

Dose.—Six globules every four hours.

Ipecacuanha, when there is much oppression of the chest; short, hurried breathing, or nausea and vomiting.

Dose.—Three globules every hour.

Sulphur, if the eruption does not appear, and the catarrhal symptoms get worse; or if there are symptoms of inflammation of the lungs.

Dose.—Four globules every two hours.

Phosphorus, if the patient is attacked in the fall or winter, and there is violent cough, with a tendency to disease of the lnngs, which if not attended to may end in pneumonia.

Dose.—Four globules every two hours.

Dulcamara, if the patient has been exposed to dampness and wet, or to a draft of air, and there is retrocession of the eruption.

Dose.—Four globules every hour.

CHICKEN POX; OR VARICELLA.

This disease bears some resemblance to small-pox. In small-pox the eruption does not appear until the third day after the fever commences; whereas, in varicella it mostly appears in the space of twenty-four hours.

This disease is mostly preceded by slight fever, nausea, and occasionally vomiting, and mostly disappears in five or six days; being generally mild in character, it seldom requires medical treatment.

REMEDIES. *Aconite*, *Belladonna*, *Coffea*, *Mercurius vivus*, *Tartar emetic*, and *Antimonium crudum*.

Aconite, during the febrile stage, will be found very serviceable.

Dose.—Four globules every three hours.

Belladonna, if with the fever there is flushing of the face, or a great deal of headache.

Dose.—Three globules every two hours.

Coffea, where there is much anxiety and restlessness, with tossing about.

Dose.—The same as Belladonna.

Mercurius vivus, if there is sore throat and considerable eruption, with the matter in the pustules turning yellow.

Dose.—Six globules every four hours.

Tartar emetic will be useful if the eruption is slow in making its appearance, or if convulsions are present.

Dose.—Six globules every two hours.

VARIOLOID.

This disease is a modified form of small-pox, and attacks those who are partially protected by vaccination, or inocculation. The fever is less severe, and shorter in duration, and the eruption comes out earlier than in genuine small-pox; begins to dry away in five or six days, finally leaves without any secondary fever, and seldom leaves any pits on the skin.

The diet should consist of light, nutritious food, and the room be kept of a regular temperature, but not too warm.

REMEDIES. *Aconite*, *Bryonia*, *Sulphur*, *Rhus toxicodendron*, and *Antimonium crudum*.

Aconite, in the commencement, will serve to allay the febrile irritation and headache.

Dose.—Four globules every two hours; or it may be given in alternation with Bryonia or Rhus toxicodendron, for the pain in the back.

Sulphur will be useful to promote the maturation of the pustules.

Dose.—Six globules three times a day.

Rhus toxicodendron, if the eruption is filled with a watery fluid, and transparent.

Dose.—The same as Aconite.

Antimonium crudum, if there is much itching of the surface. In severe cases the treatment is similar to that of small-pox.

Dose.—Six globules every four hours.

SMALL-POX; OR VARIOLA.

This eruptive disease is propagated by contagion, and seldom attacks a person more than once. It is divided into two varieties, namely: the distinct and the confluent. The distinct is characterized by the pustules being well defined, and not running into each other. The confluent is where the pustules run together, and form one continuous mass. It is one of the most malignant and loathsome diseases to which a human being is liable.

The disease mostly commences with chilliness and shuddering, after which fever follows, then headache, pain in the back and loins, weariness, with oppression of the chest, and pain in the pit of the stomach, especially upon pressure.

The period of incubation, or the length of time that elapses from exposure to the contagion until the commencement of the fever, is generally about twelve days. The fever and other premonitory symptoms continue two or three days, when the eruption, in the form of small, red spots, begins to make its appearance.

Previous to the eruption the skin is dry and hot, with much thirst; pain in the back; headache, sometimes even to delirium. The eyes are very sensitive to light, and there is great prostration of strength. During the next three days the eruption grows larger and forms pustules, which suppurate for three or four days more, and in the seventh or eighth day of the eruption (*i. e.*, the eleventh day of the disease) form scales, and begins to dry up; but as new pustules are continually making their appearance during the first three days of the eruption, and each pustule has to run through a definite course; the stage of maturation may be said to last three days longer, so that desiccation is fully established on the fourteenth day of the disease.

The eruption commences with small, red pimples—first on the face and forehead, then on the breast, body, limbs, and lastly, on the feet—somewhat similar to measles. They soon become more elevated, and upon examination are found to contain small granules, like millet-seed, distinguishing this, in the early stages, from measles and other eruptive diseases. As soon as the eruption has made its appearance, the fever abates in the distinct variety, and the patient feels better.

On the third or fourth day, when the pustules begin to fill, the tops become flattened, and as they pass on to maturity, a depression is observed in the centre. At first they contain a whitish lymph, which afterward turns yellow, and many of them burst.

Finally the pustules dry up, scabs form and begin to fall off in the order in which the eruption made its appearance—first from the face, breast, &c.—leaving the skin spotted over with pits of a reddish brown color.

During the treatment care should be taken to have the room well ventilated, and not kept too warm, nor too light. The sheets and clothing should be changed frequently, and the patient kept from scratching, in order to prevent pitting as far as possible. Some have recommended the pustules to be opened to prevent ulceration and pitting.

If there is truth in the old adage, "an ounce of prevention is better than a pound of cure," every infant should be vaccinated, and every adult re-vaccinated.

REMEDIES. *Aconite*, *Belladonna*, *Coffea*, *Chamomilla*, *Bryonia*, *Ipecacuanha*, *Tartar emetic*, *Mercurius vivus*, *Rhus toxicodendron*, *Pulsatilla*, *Stramonium*, and *Sulphur*.

Aconite is always called for in the febrile stage of this disease, if there is headache, sleepiness, eyes injected, bleeding of the nose, and if there is congestion to the internal viscera, aching in the limbs, &c.

Dose.—Six globules every two hours.

Belladonna, if there is delirium during the first

stage, with flushed face, eyes very sensitive to the light, noise intolerable, great thirst, nausea, and vomiting; or if the pustules are too red during the eruptive stage.

Dose.—Three globules every hour.

Coffea, if during the febrile stage there is much excitability and restlessness.

Dose.—Four globules every three hours.

Chamomilla will be found useful in children where there is diarrhœa or vomiting; or if there are convulsions previous to the appearance of the eruption.

Dose.—Four globules every two hours.

Bryonia will assist in bringing out the eruption; or if there is much backache, headache, or gastric disturbance, or cough, with soreness of the chest.

Dose.—Six globules every three hours.

Ipecacuanha, where there is vomiting and nausea, with oppression of the chest, before the eruption makes its appearance.

Dose.—Three globules every hour.

Tartar emetic, if the disease is preceded by convulsions, and there is drowsiness, clamminess of the skin, or sickness of the stomach.

Dose.—Dissolve a grain of the first trituration in twelve teaspoonsful of water, and give a teaspoonful every hour.

Mercurius vivus, if there is soreness of the throat; difficulty of swallowing; eyes and nose sore; breath fetid; salivation; tenderness of the stomach, with sweat and diarrhœa.

Dose.—Six globules every three hours.

Rhus toxicodendron is important during the eruptive stage, when there are acute pains in the back and loins—worse during rest—somewhat relieved by motion.

Dose.—Six globules every four hours.

Pulsatilla, if there is a disposition in the pustules to become confluent, accompanied with nausea and vomiting—worse toward night.

Dose.—Three globules every two hours.

Stramonium, if there is delirium before the eruption appears, and if the pustules do not fill properly.

Dose.—Four globules every two hours.

Sulphur, when the eruption is slow in coming out, and the pustules slow about filling; and also to alleviate the intense itching which sometimes attends the disease, especially during the drying stage.

Dose.—Four globules every three hours.

CYNANCHE TRACHEALIS; OR CROUP.

This disease is chiefly confined to early childhood, although occasionally it attacks persons more advanced in years. In sudden attacks and in severe cases it requires prompt treatment, in order to avert the danger. It may terminate fatally in twenty-four hours, but death does not generally take place before the fourth or fifth day.

Croup generally comes on with the symptoms of common cold: such as chilliness, cough, sneezing and hoarseness, which is soon followed by more or less fever; the respiration becomes hurried, with a rattling or whistling sound, and there is soreness of the windpipe. The cough, which is at first hoarse, assumes a croaking, barking tone, resembling the crowing of a young cock, or the barking of a dog.

As the danger increases, inhalation becomes more difficult, the face becomes livid, the head is thrown back, the voice sinks to a whisper, the pulse is very frequent, the pupils dilate, clammy perspiration covers the head and face, with coldness of the extremities, and death closes the scene.

We often see whole families of children, in whom there is a constitutional predisposition to this disease. When this is the case, a small amount of exposure to cold or dampness, change in dress, or in some instances derangement of the digestive organs from improper articles of food, will be sufficient to provoke an attack. A common provoking cause of croup, is the habit of sending children out to take the air about half-clothed, to show off their bare necks and fine limbs.

There are two principal varieties of croup, viz: the spasmodic, and the membranous; the latter is by far the most dangerous. It consists of a peculiar inflammation of the larynx and windpipe, causing the mucous membrane lining those parts to throw out a viscid substance, which closely adheres to the internal surface, and forms an adventitious membrane, which in fatal cases blocks up the air passages, and produces a comatose state of the brain, with symptoms of strangulation and death. In some cases, the false membrane is discharged, and the patient recovers.

REMEDIES. *Aconite*, *Tartar emetic*, *Spongia*, *Hepar sulphur*, *Ipecacuanha*, *Bryonia, Chamomilla, Phosphorus*, *Arsenicum*, *Sambucus*, *Kali bichromicum*, *Bromine*, *Iodine*, and *Mercurius iodatus.*

Aconite will be of benefit in the first stage of this disease, where the inflammatory symptoms run high, with much fever, thirst, dry skin, short dry cough, laborious breathing, &c. It is almost specific in common catarrhal croup.

Dose.—Dissolve thirty globules in half a tumbler of water, and give a teaspoonful every twenty or thirty minutes, according to the violence of the symptoms, until the patient is better.

Tartar emetic may be used, where the attack comes on suddenly at night; with a choking cough or an accumulation of mucus in the throat, with hurried breathing, hoarse hollow cough, &c.

Dose.—Dissolve a grain of the first trituration in a tumbler half full of water, and give a teaspoonful every fifteen or twenty minutes, until the symptoms are relieved, and then not so often.

Spongia, if the skin has become moist, the breathing somewhat easier, and the paroxysms of cough a little lighter, but still the grating and wheezing sound of respiration remaining.

Dose.—Six globules every one or two hours.

Hepar sulphur, when perspiration has taken place, the breathing easier, but still the cough is dry and hollow, and there is mucus rattling in the throat, with hoarseness.

Dose.—The same as of Tartar emetic, only at longer intervals—from two to four hours.

Ipecacuanha may be given in alternation with Aconite, where there is a constant disposition to vomit; cough, especially at night, with stiffness of the body, and bluish face, or loss of breath with the least motion.

Dose.—Three globules every hour.

Bryonia, spasmodic and suffocating cough, with oppression and rattling in the chest, difficult swallowing, with great dryness in the throat, increased by the least motion.

Dose.—Four globules every two hours.

Chamomilla, dry cough, worse at night, with accumulation of mucus in the throat; continual tickling in the throat, with wheezing in the chest during sleep.

Dose.—Four globules every two hours.

Phosphorus, dry tickling cough, with hoarseness and pain in the chest, as if excoriated; or expectoration of mucus, with hollow cough.

Dose.—Six globules every three hours.

Arsenicum, dry cough, worse on lying down, with difficult breathing and accumulation of tenacious mucus in the larynx, or expectoration of bloody mucus.

Dose.—Six globules every four hours.

Sambucus, suffocating cough at night, with puffed bluish face; starting in the sleep, with profuse perspiration at night.

Dose.—Four globules every two hours.

Kali bichromicun, *Bromine*, and *Iodine*. These remedies have of late been highly recommended in croup, especially in cases where there is a predisposition to the formation of the false membrane, and where there is a copious secretion of mucus, and ineffectual efforts to expectorate.

Dose.—Six globules of either, every one, two, or three hours, as the case may require.

Mercurius iodatus, where there is salivation, and a constant tendency to inflammation of the throat, with ulceration, and enlargement of the tonsils.

Dose.—A grain of the third trituration every two or three hours.

ASTHMA OF MILLAR.

This affection is generally known by the name of "spasmodic croup." The attack is apt to come on suddenly, and in the night. The child wakes up with difficulty in getting its breath; causing a cooing kind of noise, with a dry, harsh, half-suppressed cough. In severe cases, the face becomes somewhat livid and swollen, the countenance expresses the greatest anxiety, and the child is evidently afraid of suffocation. The disease is chiefly confined to young children of delicate constitution, and is generally brought on by exposure.

REMEDIES. *Aconite*, *Ipecacuanha*, *Arsenicum*, *Sambucus*, and *Pulsatilla*.

Aconite, if it comes on suddenly at night, with a suffocating cough; hoarse voice; respiration short and anxious, with fever; is specific.

Dose.—Six globules every half hour, or hour.

Ipecacuanha, if there is oppression of the chest, with accumulation of mucus; rattling in the windpipe; short anxious breathing; pale face, with coldness of the extremities.

Dose.—Six globules every hour.

Arsenicum, in violent attacks of asthma, from catarrhal oppression; prostration of strength; great anguish, with cold perspiration; and the symptoms aggravated between midnight and daylight.

Dose.—Six globules every hour.

Sambucus, if the attack comes on suddenly, with dry, hollow cough and fear of suffocation; anxious tossing about, and inability to sleep.

Dose.—Three globules every hour.

Pulsatilla, cough, with constriction of the larynx; worse at night; increased by lying down, with a desire to vomit, and difficult expectoration of mucus.

Dose.—Six globules every hour.

PURTUSSIS; OR HOOPING-COUGH.

Hooping-cough generally begins with the symptoms of common cold. In about a week the catarrhal symptoms disappear, except the cough, which increases in severity, and returns in paroxysms every two or three hours. The quantity of mucus in the throat and chest increases, and, in a few days more, the characteristic noise, called hooping, makes its appearance. If a spell of coughing occurs soon after a meal, vomiting is apt to follow the paroxysm. Bleeding of the nose is also a frequent attendant upon hooping-cough.

REMEDIES. *Aconite*, *Drosera*, *Cuprum metallicum*, *Dulcamara*, *Pulsatilla*, *Nux vomica*, *Ipecacuanha*, *Belladonna*, *Cina*, *Conium maculatum*, *Mercurius vivus*, *Phosphorus*, and *Bryonia alba*.

Aconite, in the very commencement of the disease, if there is febrile excitement, with dry whistling cough, causing a burning pain in the larynx, worse on coughing.

Dose.—Six globules four times a day.

Drosera, if the patient is worse during rest; warm perspiration at night; chills, without thirst; also when the cough is loud and hoarse, and the paroxysms violent.

Dose.—Six globules night and morning.

Cuprum metallicum in violent cases, especially where the breathing is suspended during the attack of coughing; rigidity of the patient; vomiting on the return of respiration, and slow breathing afterward.

Dose.—Four globules after each paroxysm.

Dulcamara may be used, if the attack is brought

on by exposure to cold and dampness, with hoarseness, loose cough, and copious expectoration.

Dose.—Six globules every four hours.

Pulsatilla, for a disposition to vomit after each paroxysm, with loose cough; sneezing; weakness of the eyes; increased watery discharge from the eyes, and hoarseness.

Dose.—Four globules three times a day.

Nux vomica, if there is great anguish, with dry cough; blueness of the face, with dread of suffocation—worse after midnight; with bleeding of the nose, and vomiting.

Dose.—Six globules twice a day.

Ipecacuánha, if there is vomiting, and the cough is dry and spasmodic, without wheezing; apparent danger of suffocation, with blueness of the face.

Dose.—Six globules every four hours.

Belladonna, if in the commencement there is a dry, barking, hollow cough, which is worse at night, accompanied with congestion to the head; sneezing; bleeding at the nose; blood-shot eyes; soreness of the throat, with difficulty in swallowing liquids.

Dose.—Six globules every six or eight hours, according to circumstances.

Cina, if on coughing, there is rigidity of the body; bleeding from the mouth and nose; or if there are symptoms of worms present—as picking of the nose, griping pain in the bowels, or itching of the anus.

Dose.—Six globules twice a day.

Conium maculatum, if the paroxysms are very severe, and are apt to occur at night, accompanied or followed by vomiting.

Dose.—Six globules three times a day.

Mercurius vivus, if there is a succession of paroxysms of coughing, especially at night, after which there is a considerable interval of rest; or dry cough, with watery coryza, which excoriates the nose.

Dose.—Six globules twice a day.

Phosphorus, if the cough is severe, hoarse, and dry; croupy, or there is loss of the voice; the cough causing headache; and if there is difficulty and pain on breathing, with other symptoms, threatening disease of the lungs.

Dose.—Six globules three times a day.

Bryonia, if there is oppression of the chest, with hoarseness; dry spasmodic cough, worse in the evening, and after eating and drinking, with vomiting of food; dryness of the throat, with diffi culty of swallowing.

Dose.—Six globules night and morning.

HYDROCEPHALUS; OR DROPSY OF THE HEAD.

This disease is mostly confined to children between the ages of six months and seven years. Those with large heads, slowly closing fontanelles, and those of a scrofulous taint, are most liable to be attacked. In the commencement, the diagnosis is sometimes obscure; as it may be taken for worm fever, disordered stomach, or from teething, &c. Among the most prominent symptoms are: headache; stupor; nausea and vomiting; constipation of the bowels; convulsions; rolling of the head; staring look; dilatation of the pupils; pulse varying—at times frequent, and again very slow.

REMEDIES. *Aconite*, *Belladonna*, *Bryonia*, *Helleborus*, *Mercurius*, *Cuprum aceticum*, *Sulphur*, *Opium*, and *Zincum metalicum*.

Aconite in the commencement, when there is much fever; dry and hot skin, and quick pulse.

Dose.—Four globules every two hours.

Belladonna, if there is congestion, with heat of the head and delirium; red, bloated face; throbbing of the arteries of the neck; dilated pupils, and dread of light.

Dose.—Four globules every two hours.

Bryonia, confusion of the head; giddiness, especially on raising the head; throbbing in the head; face red and swollen; great thirst; eyes convulsed and fixed; constipation, with distended abdomen; urine suppressed, and difficult respiration.

Dose.—Four globules every two hours.

Helleborus in the acute and chronic stages, where there is confusion, dullness, and heaviness in the head, with burning heat—the head thrown backward, with convulsive movements of the limbs. It is especially recommended where the disease follows measles or scarlatina.

Dose.—Six globules every hour until better, and then not so often.

Mercurius, if there is looseness of the bowels; dull and stupid feeling, with weakness of memory; or feeling of intoxication, with redness and swelling of the face. Suitable after Belladonna.

Dose.—Six globules every two hours.

Cuprum aceticum, if it arise from suppressed eruptions, with convulsions and congestion to the head; throbbing in the temples; headache, with great weakness; disturbed sleep; flushed face; nausea and vomiting; quick, full pulse, and worse toward night.

Dose.—Four globules every hour.

Sulphur is useful where there is more excitement than torpidity of the brain; also in the inflammatory stage after Aconite or Belladonna.

Dose.—Three globules every four hours.

Opium, if there are convulsions, with loss of consciousness; coma; delirium; startling visions; frightful dreams, with fixed eyes and stertorous breathing.

Dose.—Four globules every hour.

Zincum metallicum, if there is threatened paralysis of the brain, with involuntary discharge of fæces; coldness of the skin; quick pulse, &c.

Dose.—Six globules every one or two hours.

SCROFULA.

This very common disease is found in all classes and in all ages, but more frequently in young persons than in those of maturer years.

The peculiar diathesis is generally transmitted from parent to child by hereditary influence, and is manifested by the fairness of the skin, large size of the head, prominence of the abdomen, enlargement of the joints, smallness and laxity of the muscles, with a prevailing tendency to looseness of the bowels. It is more common among colored children than with white.

The symptoms which indicate the presence of scrofula are: thickening of the eye-lids, slight inflammation of the nostrils, enlargement of the lymphatic glands on the sides of the neck, or similar enlargement of the like glands under the arms and in the groins. At first they are hard, and moveable under the skin, withvery little sensibility. They may continue in this state for years, and finally disappear; but such is not generally the case, for they mostly become larger, more painful, the skin reddens, suppuration is established, and scrofulous ulcers are formed. The matter discharged is thin, and mixed with portions of a curdled substance resembling cheese.

REMEDIES. *Mercurius vivus*, *Dulcamara*, *Belladonna*, *Calcarea carbonica*, *Sulphur*, *Graphites*, *Hepar sulphur*, *Silicea*, *Mercurius iodatus*, and *Arsenicum*.

Mercurius vivus, in inflammation and swelling of the glands of the throat, with difficulty of swallowing; enlargement and suppuration of inguinal glands, with discharge of a yellow, curdy matter.

Dose.—Six globules night and morning.

Dulcamara is suited to persons of a leucophlegmatic temperament, with irritable disposition, and where the glands harden and inflame with the least attack of cold.

Dose.—Six globules twice a day.

Belladonna, inflammation and suppuration of the glands, with dryness of the mouth; frequent soreness of the throat; swelling of the tonsils, and difficulty of swallowing.

Dose.—Six globules three times a day.

Calcarea carbonica, hardness and suppuration of the glands; swelling of the mesenteric glands; large head and open fontanelles; prominent abdomen; pale and bloated face, with constipation or diarrhœa.

Dose.—Six globules night and morning.

Sulphur, swelling, suppuration, or ulceration of the glands; loose, spongy, and flabby flesh; disposition to take cold; profuse perspiration, with pale and bloated face.

Dose.—Six globules night and morning.

Graphites, swelling, suppuration, and induration of the glands; obstinate scrofulous ulcers; inflammation and ulceration of the eye-lids; paleness of the face, with swelling of the tonsils and difficult deglutition.

Dose.—Six globules twice a day.

Hepar sulphur, pale and bloated face, with induration and suppuration of the glands; also where there is a disposition to ulceration, soreness and swelling of the throat.

Dose.—Six globules three times a day.

Silicea will be useful in all glandular enlargements; suppuration, with ichorous discharge of a yellowish color and fetid odor; also in agglutination of the eye-lids.

Dose.—Six globules every night.

Mercurius iodatus, in swelling and inflammation of the glands of the throat, with difficult deglutition.

Dose.—One grain of the first trituration daily.

Arsenicum, emaciation; swelling of the glands of the neck; bloated face; hard and distended abdomen, with diarrhœa and debility, especially if the child eat meat greedily.

Dose.—Four globules three times a day.

WORMS; OR WORM FEVER.

The presence of worms in the alimentary canal mostly arises from a diseased state of the mucous membrane lining the canal, constitutional peculiarity, or hereditary predisposition.

The most prominent symptoms indicating their presence are: pains in the abdomen, especially in the umbilical region, being mostly a sensation of pressure, at times so violent as to resemble colic; itching of the nose and anus, especially at night; paleness of the countenance; livid circles around the eyes; fetid breath; irregular appetite frequent starts, and fright during sleep; bleeding of the nose, &c.

REMEDIES. *Cina*, *China*, *Belladonna*, *Spigelia*, *Santonin*, *Mercurius vivus*, *Ipecacuanha*, *Pulsatilla*, and *Nux vomica*.

Cina, if there is chilliness; hard and frequent pulse; disturbed sleep; ill humor; itching of the nose and anus; vomiting; hot and distended abdomen, with colicky pains.

Dose.—Six globules night and morning.

China, where there is fullness of the abdomen; heartburn; spasmodic action of the muscles; retching; sensitiveness of the nervous system, and aggravation of the symptoms at night.

Dose.—Six globules every night before going to bed, in a teaspoonful of water.

Belladonna, if there is starting in the sleep; great thirst; spasms; congestion toward the brain, and involuntary discharge of fæces and urine.

Dose.—Four globules three times a day.

Spigelia, where there is pinching pain in the abdomen; diarrhœa; paleness of countenance; itching of the nose, and palpitation of the heart.

Dose.—Six globules in a teaspoonful of water night and morning.

Santonin, where there is much itching of the nose and anus; restlessness; irritable mood; pain in the abdomen, with colic.

Dose.—One grain of the third trituration, night and morning until better.

Mercurius vivus, where there is diarrhœic stools; distension of the abdomen; increased secretion of saliva in the mouth; itching and soreness of the anus, with discharge of worms.

Dose.—Six globules in a teaspoonful of water night and morning.

Ipecacuanha, if there are griping pains in the abdomen; vomiting of large quantities of mucus; aversion to food; emaciation, with creeping and itching of the anus.

Dose.—Six globules night and morning until better.

Pulsatilla, if the face is pale; bad smell from the mouth; nausea, with disposition to vomit; sour or bitter eructations; distension of the abdomen; stools loose and mixed with mucus, and soreness of the anus.

Dose.—The same as of Ipecacuanha.

Nux vomica, if there is continual itching of the nose; dullness of the head; irritable mood; aversion to food and drinks; cutting pain in the abdomen; constipation; creeping in the anus and rectum, and discharge of worms from the anus.

Dose.—Six globules every night on going to bed, in a teaspoonful of water until better.

MUMPS; OR PAROTITIS.

This disease is chiefly incident to childhood, and occurs but once. It is most prone to take place in cold, damp, and changeable weather, and consists of an inflammatory swelling of the parotid glands (one or both) which are situated near the angle of the lower jaw, just below the ear. The inflammation sometimes attains a very high degree, and extends to the throat and tonsils, causing great difficulty in swallowing, and even threatens suffocation. It is usually ushered in by chilliness, nausea, and other symptoms of cold; but the swelling soon after makes its appearance, and reveals the true nature of the disease.

When the disease occurs in adults, metastasis is liable to take place in the breasts of females, and in the testicles of males, from exposure to cold or dampness, and from repelling applications made to the swollen glands.

The patient should be kept warm, and protected from the liability of taking cold.

REMEDIES. *Mercurius vivus*, *Belladonna*, *Carbo vegetabilis*, *Hyoscyamus*, *Cocculus*, *Nux vomica*, and *Pulsatilla*.

Mercurius vivus, if it is atttended with much

pain; the glands much swollen and inflamed, with stinging and throbbing, or with intense redness; beating and stinging pain on swallowing; worse when taking dry food, than when taking liquids.

Dose.—Six globules every three or four hours until better, then administer six globules night and morning, until all the symptoms disappear.

Belladonna will be useful, if the swelling is red, or assumes an erysipelatous appearance, with difficulty in swallowing; or if there is a sudden disappearance of the redness and swelling, threatening metastasis to the brain—which is attended with unconsciousness and delirium.

Dose.—Dissolve eight globules in a tumbler half full of water, and give a teaspoonful of the solution every one or two hours, according to the severity of the symptoms.

Carbo vegetabilis, if the tumor is hard, accompanied with slow fever; voice very hoarse; or if there has been cold taken, from want of care.

Dose.—Six globules every four hours.

Hyoscyamus, if there is constriction of the throat, with difficulty in swallowing; loss of speech; staring and distorted eyes. It is especially useful after Belladonna, when that remedy has failed to afford relief.

Dose.—The same as directed for Belladonna.

Cocculus, if there is digging pain in the lower jaw; spasms in the stomach; dryness of the throat and mouth, with lacerating pain in the swollen gland.

Dose.—The same as directed for Carbo vegetabilis.

If there is metastasis to the breasts or testicles, give Nux vomica or Pulsatilla, and apply flannels, wrung out of hot water, to the original seat of the disease.

Dose.—Six globules every four hours.

SORE-THROAT OR QUINSY.

This disease consists of an inflammatory swelling of the throat and tonsils, which become enlarged and assume a florid hue, accompanied with fever, painful deglutition, hoarseness, heat, and darting pains in the throat. It is often caused by getting the feet wet, exposure to a draft of air, sitting in damp clothes, or sudden changes of temperature, producing a check of perspiration.

REMEDIES *Aconite*, *Belladonna*, *Mercurius vivus*, *Chamomilla*, *Dulcamara*, *Bryonia*, *Nux vomica*, *Hepar sulphur*, *Arsenicum*, and *Pulsatilla*.

Aconite in the commencement, where there is much fever; inflammation, and dark red appearance of the tonsils; scraping in the throat, with almost inability to swallow.

Dose.—Dissolve twelve globules in a wineglassful of water, and take a teaspoonful every two hours until better.

Belladonna, violent burning in the throat, with fever; soreness of the throat when swallowing; inability to swallow liquids; bright redness of the throat and tonsils, with swelling; violent headache, and determination of blood to the head.

Dose.—Six globules every four hours, either dry upon the tongue or in a spoonful of water.

Mercurius vivus, if the inflammation is bright red, and very painful; excoriating pain in the throat, especially in swallowing, with constant desire to swallow, and almost inability to do so—especially drinks, which are returned through the nose—and profuse accumulation of saliva in the mouth.

Dose.—Six globules every four hours until better.

Chamomilla is especially suited to children, where the attack was brought on by a sudden check of perspiration; the glands of the neck are painful and swollen; difficulty of swallowing, as if something was lodged in the throat; hoarseness; fever in the evening, with heat alternating with chilliness.

Dose.—Four globules in a teaspoonful of water every two or three hours.

Dulcamara, if the attack was brought on by getting wet; or comes on in damp, changeable weather.

Dose.—The same as directed for Aconite.

Bryonia, sore throat, with hoarseness, and difficulty of swallowing; dry cough with difficult respiration; dryness of the throat, with shootings in it on being touched; constipation, especially if the attack was brought on by sudden suppression of perspiration, or from drinking ice-water.

Dose.—Four globules in a teaspoonful of water every two or three hours.

Nux vomica, soreness and rawness of the throat, as if swollen, especially on swallowing, as if there was a plug in the throat; swelling of the tonsils; small, fetid ulcers in the mouth; constipation.

Dose.—Six globules every four hours.

Hepar sulphur, if the disease has made rapid progress, and suppuration has commenced. It will be valuable in bringing about the discharge of matter, so as to relieve the patient as quickly as possible.

Dose.—Six globules every two hours in a teaspoonful of water.

Arsenicum, if there are ulcers with hard, raised edges, and shining, red areola; breath putrid and offensive; tongue foul; loss of strength; burning heat, and great restlessness.

Dose.—Three globules in a spoonful of water every two or three hours.

Pulsatilla, scraping and raw feeling in the throat, as if swollen, without thirst; difficulty of swallowing, as if the throat were narrower than usual—the swollen glands are painful to the touch.

Dose.—The same as directed for Nux vomica.

DYSENTERY.

The seasons of the year in which this disease is most prevalent, are spring and fall. The most common symptoms are: frequent desire to evacuate the bowels; constant tenesmus; violent straining, with discharge of frothy mucus, or mucus mixed with blood; and frequently pure blood, or blood and matter, sometimes resembling shreds, like the scraping of the intestines. It generally commences with chilliness, afterward heat; thirst; disposition to vomit; pulse accelerated; and is sometimes preceded by diarrhœa—it is mostly caused by taking cold, errors in diet, sudden check of perspiration, unripe fruit, noxious vapors from marshy districts, &c.

REMEDIES. *Mercurius corrosivus*, *Mercurius vivus*, *Aconite*, *Ipecacuanha*, *Chamomilla*, *Rhus toxicodendron*, *Bryonia*, *Nux vomica*, *Colocynthis*, *Arsenicum*, and *Sulphur*.

Mercurius corrosivus, violent pain in the bowels;

abdomen painful to the touch; griping or cutting in the abdomen; discharge of bloody mucus or pure blood, with violent colic; or ineffectual urging and tenesmus; cutting pain in the rectum.

Dose.—Six globules every two or three hours, according to the violence of the case.

Mercurius vivus, constant desire for stool, with slight discharge; bloody stools, with painful smarting sensation of the anus; black, tenacious, pitch-like stools; or dark green, bilious, and frothy stools.

Dose.—The same as directed for Mercurius corrosive.

Aconite, if there is much fever; dry, parched skin; violent thirst; pain in the limbs; frequent watery and loose stools, with tenesmus; involuntary stools, with pain in the rectum. It is especially adapted to dysenteries occurring in the fall of the year, when the weather is very changeable.

Dose.—Six globules every two or three hours until better.

Ipecacuanha, bloody stools, with cutting pain in the anus; nausea; tenesmus and colic; burning and stinging in the rectum, with desire for stool and discharge of green mucus.

Dose.—The same as directed for Aconite.

Chamomilla, if the attack was brought on by a sudden change from heat to cold, causing a check of perspiration; feverish heat, and redness of the cheeks; restlessness; discharges corrosive, and like mixed eggs.

Dose.—The same as directed for Aconite.

Rhus toxicodendron, if there are nightly evacuations, which occur involuntary, or, at an advanced stage of the disease, should typhoid symptoms set in; scarlet redness of the abdomen; stools mixed with blood; headache, and pain in all the limbs.

Dose.—Six globules in a teaspoonful of water every two or three hours.

Bryonia, if the attack has been brought about by using cold drinks, iced fruit, &c.; stools thin and bloody, with a sharp burning pain in the rectum; colic, with cutting pain in the abdomen.

Dose.—The same as directed for Rhus toxicodendron.

Nux vomica, small stools, consisting principally of blood and mucus, accompanied with urging and tenesmus of the rectum; pitch-like stools; sensation as if the rectum was contracted; burning and pricking of the hæmorrhoidal tumors at the anus.

Dose.—Six globules every two or three hours according to the urgency of the symptoms.

Colocynthis, frequent stools, with tenesmus and griping pain in the intestines, causing the patient to bend double; bloody stools; fæces consisting of undigested food; contraction of the rectum during stools, &c.

Dose.—Twelve globules dissolved in a tumbler half full of water, and a teaspoonful of the solution every fifteen or thirty minutes; or at longer intervals, according to the violence of the symptoms present.

Arsenicum, pain in the abdomen, with ineffectual urging and tenesmus; discharges acrid and burning, or very fetid; great prostration of strength, and trembling; bloody evacuations, with vomiting and excessive colic.

Dose.—Six globules in a teaspoonful of water every two or three hours.

Sulphur, discharge of blood-streaked mucus, with colic; fever, and want of appetite; tenesmus; frequent desire to stool, mostly at night; prolapsus of the rectum during stool.

Dose.—Six globules in a teaspoonful of water every three hours.

VACCINATION.

This is a purely homœopathic means of preventing one of the most loathsome diseases to which the human system is liable—the small-pox. Vaccination alone, has probably, within the last fifty years—since its general introduction—saved more human life than all other remedial means put together, have done, in twice that length of time.

It will answer well to vaccinate a child at almost any age, but probably about the sixth month is the best time, as the child is as easy nursed at that age as any other, and is less liable to get the pustule broken, from accidental causes or its own scratching, than when older.

It is a matter of great importance to obtain the virus from a healthy child of healthy parents, as few removes from the matter obtained from the cow as possible. The child selected should be free from scrofulous taint and all other hereditary diseases, especially cutaneous diseases.

The proper place to insert the matter is on the outer portion of the left arm, about half-way between the elbow and the shoulder.

To prepare the matter, take a portion of the scab and rub it up with a drop of clean water with the point of a lancet on a piece of glass or other hard and smooth substance, until it attains the consistency of cream. Then take a portion of the matter thus prepared on the point of the lancet, and insert it beneath the cuticle, by making three or four slight punctures close together; then apply more matter, and allow it to become dry without being wiped off.

If the operation is successful, on the fourth or fifth day a small red pimple is observable, which the next day becomes a little vesicle, and increases in size until it reaches about the quarter of an inch in diameter. On the seventh day the areola is formed, which goes on increasing until the ninth or tenth day, when it is about an inch and a half in diameter. The lymph contained in the vesicle is at first clear, then milky, afterward yellow, and finally dries into a mahogany brown scab, indented near the middle, with a hardened point in the centre. The constitutional symptoms usually appear about the seventh day, and consist of a little fever and restlessness, with some soreness in the axilla of the vaccinated arm—they last from twelve to eighteen hours. The scab falls off about the seventeenth day, leaving a cicatrix, with a number of small pointed pits in its inclosure.

The vaccine disease is so mild in its course, that medical treatment is seldom necessary. If the fever should be considerable, a dose or two of Aconite or Belladonna will be sufficient to remove all the unpleasant symptoms.

The best means of preventing the development of eruptions which sometimes follow vaccination, is to administer a dose of homœopathic sulphur on the evening of the eighth day.

INDEX.

THE END.

www.ingramcontent.com/pod-product-compliance
Lightning Source LLC
LaVergne TN
LVHW010249110826
845151LV00004B/1427

* 9 7 8 1 4 2 5 5 2 2 9 2 6 *